LOW IMPACT AND GENTLE CHAIR EXERCISES FOR SENIORS

LEARN CARDIO, YOGA, CORE, AND STRENGTH TRAINING TO IMPROVE ENDURANCE, BALANCE, AND FLEXIBILITY IN 20-MINUTE ROUTINES

DIANA IGRAM

CONTENTS

Introduction   5

1. THE AGING BODY AND EXERCISE   9
   The Science Behind the Change   10
   Common Issues That May Arise   32
   Other Common Issues   42
   Exercises Can Help   47
   Age Is Just a Number   52

2. WHY CHAIR EXERCISES?   55
   The Benefits of Chair Exercises   57
   Setting Fitness Goals   62
   Tips to Keep In Mind   74
   Tools Needed   77
   Staying Motivated   77
   Age Is Just a Number   81

3. CHAIR YOGA   85
   Poses for the Neck   86
   Poses for the Core and Arms   98
   Poses for Feet and Toes   122
   Age Is Just a Number   137

4. CARDIO EXERCISES   139
   Warm Up   140
   Exercises to Get the Heart Pumping   148
   Age Is Just a Number   163

5. CORE EXERCISES   165
   Age Is Just a Number   180

6. STRENGTH TRAINING   181
   Strength Training for Upper Body   182
   Strength Training for Lower Body   194
   Age Is Just a Number   203

7. 20-MINUTE ROUTINES   205
    Routine #1: All About Stretching/Yoga   206
    Routine #2: Arm Day   207
    Routine #3: Leg Day   207
    Routine #4: Core and Cardio Day   208
    Age Is Just a Number   210

8. EXERCISE LOGBOOK   211

    Conclusion   215
    References   219

INTRODUCTION

While growing older is a blessing envied by many, it comes with its fair share of issues. From the fear and anxiety of not being able to take care of yourself to unending health issues and sometimes even memory loss, aging can really take its toll on you. However, through every challenge, one thing is for sure: every senior desires to live long and healthy so they can be with their families for as long as possible. They don't want their health to deteriorate to a point where they cannot be independent, contributing members of society. I am sure you also feel this way, which is why you should read this book.

You might have already heard about low-impact chair exercises, but I want to teach you to have a holistic approach to your routines. You will benefit immensely from this book if you experience the following:

- decreased mobility, flexibility, and resistance
- reduced quality of life
- mental health concerns
- convenience or accessibility issues

In this book, you'll learn everything you need to know to get started with chair exercises immediately. From yoga/stretching to cardio, core, and strength training, you will be equipped with various workout routines. Ultimately, you will feel confident in your abilities to work out from the comfort of your home, regardless of your mobility status. You will find renewed health and wellness and start enjoying your life again.

EXPLORING THE AUTHOR'S JOURNEY

I'm a retiree who made the decision to stay active and healthy. From a young age, I embraced a wide range of exercises such as hiking, jogging, and high-impact aerobics, relishing the exhilaration they brought. As the years passed and I gracefully aged, I adjusted my routine to include low-impact and gentler exercises to accommodate my changing needs.

However, I encountered a new challenge in the past five years: chronic knee pain. This limitation in my range of motion prompted me to explore chair exercises, an alternative approach that proved to be both effective and enjoyable. Through consistent practice, I experienced the incredible benefits of these exercises first-hand, not only in terms of physical well-being but also in maintaining a positive mindset.

With an unwavering belief that an active lifestyle holds the key to happiness and longevity, I now yearn to share my wisdom with others. I'm determined to help individuals from all walks of life, especially those who face physical constraints or prefer the comfort of their own homes. The idea of a book was born—an all-encompassing resource that individuals could turn to, unlocking improved health and wellness within the confines of their own living spaces.

Drawing from my wealth of personal experience, I have set out to put pen to paper, capturing my insights, techniques, and guidance. This book will serve as a trusted companion for those seeking to embrace an active lifestyle, even when mobility is limited. Through clear and accessible instructions, my goal is to empower and enable you to embark on your own journey toward enhanced physical and mental well-being.

This will be an easy-to-read manual focusing on fitness and leading fulfilling lives through small daily lifestyle changes. By sharing my expertise, I hope to instill confidence, motivation, and a sense of possibility in those who may feel discouraged or constrained by their circumstances. It's my desire to create a ripple effect that fosters a community of individuals who believe that age should never be a barrier to leading an active, fulfilling life.

So, join me in this extraordinary endeavor as I open the doors to a world of chair exercises where health, happiness, and vitality await.

Revitalize Your Health and Mobility: Embrace the Power of Chair Exercises for Seniors Today!

I assure you, this book is not a get-healthy-quick scheme. Rather, it focuses on small daily changes that will slowly but surely become habits. Please note that although chair exercises are a holistic approach to health and longevity, they do not substitute a medical doctor's expertise or prescription. Rather, they work hand-in-hand with your medicine unless or until you're told otherwise by your physician. Finally, let me ask you this: Do chair exercises have the power to enhance a senior's physical, mental, emotional, and spiritual well-being? The answer is simple—they sure do! If you're wondering how, it's time to find out.

1

THE AGING BODY AND EXERCISE

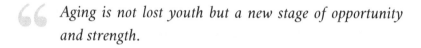 *Aging is not lost youth but a new stage of opportunity and strength.*

— BETTY FRIEDAN

One minute you are young, energetic, and adventurous, and the next, you can barely do a squat to save your life. Well, I don't want to project, but the change really was that random and drastic for me. However, while my body changed, my mind didn't keep up with it. I was still me; I still wanted to go hiking with my family, enjoy an intense session of aerobics, and go for my morning jog.

The truth of the matter is that our bodies change as we age. It's scientific, and there's no running away from it. But that doesn't mean that we should stop enjoying our lives or taking care of our physical, mental, and emotional well-being. On the contrary, we need to focus on self-care now more than ever.

THE SCIENCE BEHIND THE CHANGE

As we age, both individual cells and entire organs undergo transformations, leading to changes in both functionality and physical appearance. Perhaps it's crucial to understand these changes extensively to realize how low-impact and gentle chair exercises can change our lives as seniors. Let's get right into it (Stefanacci, 2022):

Aging Cells

With age, our cells begin to function less effectively. With time, these cells die. There's nothing wrong with that; it's just another normal part of how our bodies work.

There are various factors that lead to the death of old cells. First, they die due to apoptosis, a process programmed by the genes of cells. You can think of this process as cell suicide, which is triggered by the aging of cells, among other things. It's necessary for old cells to die so that room is created for new ones. Having too many cells may also trigger this program.

Additionally, old cells die because they have a finite number of divisions they can undergo. This limitation is determined by our genes. When a cell reaches its division limit, it grows larger, persists for a period, and eventually perishes. This restriction on cell division involves a component known as a telomere, which helps in the movement of genetic material during cell division. With every cell division, the telomeres slowly become shorter, and with time, it gets too short for any further division. The cell will ultimately deteriorate.

At times, cell death occurs directly due to damage from radiation, sunlight, and chemotherapy drugs. They can also suffer damage from specific by-products generated during their regular functions.

Aging Organs

Your organs function best when the cells within them are fully functional. However, as cells age, their functionality tends to decline. Additionally, in certain organs, cells die and are not replaced, leading to a decrease in cell numbers. The testes, ovaries, liver, and kidneys are notable examples where the number of cells significantly diminishes with age. When the cell count drops too low, an organ's ability to function normally is compromised. Consequently, most organs exhibit reduced functionality as individuals grow older.

However, it's important to note that not all organs experience substantial cell loss. The brain, for instance, is relatively spared in healthy older individuals, with minimal loss of brain cells. Significant cell loss is prevalent in people who have suffered a stroke and those with neurodegenerative disorders (Alzheimer's or Parkinson's disease).

The musculoskeletal system is often one of the first areas to show signs of aging. Changes in the eyes typically occur early in mid-life, followed by changes in the ears. As we age, most internal functions experience a decline. Generally, bodily functions reach their peak around the age of 30 and then gradually decrease over time.

However, despite this decline, most functions remain sufficient because our organs typically begin with a much greater functional capacity than the body actually requires (known as functional reserve). If, for instance, half of your liver is damaged, the remaining healthy tissue is quite capable of maintaining normal function. Therefore, disorders usually account for the majority of functional decline in old age rather than the natural aging process itself. Your body is now much less equipped to deal with extreme temperature fluctuations, intense physical activities, and certain disorders. You're also more prone to drug/medicine-induced side effects. Your heart, kidneys, brain, blood vessels, and urinary organs are more prone to malfunction under stress compared to the rest of your organs.

Bones and Joints

You have probably already come across the word osteopenia, which refers to the moderate reduction of bone density. Severe loss of bone density, however, is referred to as osteoporosis. As we age, our bones undergo changes that can lead to decreased density. Whether the decrease is moderate or severe will determine the problems you'll encounter.

Osteoporosis makes bones weaker and more susceptible to fractures. In women, the loss of bone density accelerates after menopause due to reduced estrogen production, a hormone that plays a crucial role in preventing the excessive breakdown of bone during the body's natural process of bone formation, breakdown, and reformation.

The decrease in bone density is partially attributed to reduced calcium content, which contributes to bone strength. The body absorbs less calcium from food, leading to lower calcium levels. Additionally, there is a slight decrease in vitamin D levels, which is necessary for the body to utilize calcium effectively. Certain bones are more affected by this decline. The hip's thighbone (femur) end, the wrist's arm bones (radius and ulna), and the spinal bones (vertebrae) are particularly vulnerable.

Moreover, the vertebrae at the top of the spine undergo changes that can cause the head to tilt forward, resulting in the compression of the throat. This can lead to difficulties in swallowing and an increased risk of choking. The vertebrae themselves become less dense, and the cushions of tissue between them, known as discs, lose fluid and become thinner. Consequently, the spine gradually becomes shorter, contributing to the overall height reduction experienced by older individuals.

Over time, the cartilage that covers the joints tends to become thinner, primarily due to the accumulated wear and tear from years of movement. As a result, the surfaces of the joints may not glide over each other as smoothly as they did before, making the joint slightly more prone to injury. Prolonged use of joints or repeated injuries can cause damage to the cartilage, leading to a common age-related disorder known as osteoarthritis. This condition, characterized by the deterioration of cartilage, is frequently observed in the later stages of life.

With age, ligaments that hold joints together and tendons that connect muscles to bones tend to lose elasticity, resulting in a sensation of tightness or stiffness in the joints. These tissues also weaken over time, leading to a decrease in overall flexibility for most individuals. Ligaments and tendons become more prone to tearing, and when injuries occur, the healing process tends to be slower. These changes happen due to a reduction in the activity of the cells responsible for maintaining ligaments and tendons.

Blood Production

As we age, the quantity of active bone marrow, which is responsible for producing blood cells, diminishes. Consequently, there is a reduction in the production of blood cells. However, in most cases, the bone marrow is still able to generate an adequate amount of blood cells throughout a person's lifetime.

Challenges may arise when there is a significant increase in the demand for blood cells, such as during the development of anemia, infection, or instances of bleeding. In such situations, the bone marrow faces limitations in its ability to ramp up blood cell production in response to the body's requirements.

Brain and Nervous System

As we age, it's common for the number of nerve cells in the brain to decrease, but the brain possesses certain mechanisms to partially make up for this loss:

- As cells are lost, the remaining nerve cells establish new connections among themselves.
- In certain regions of the brain, new nerve cells can continue to form even during old age.
- The brain exhibits redundancy, meaning it has more cells than necessary for most activities.

The levels of chemical substances involved in transmitting messages within the brain generally decrease with age, although some may increase. Additionally, nerve cells can experience a reduction in the number of receptors available to receive these chemical messages. Blood flow to the brain also diminishes. These age-related changes may result in a slight decline in brain function. Older individuals may react and perform tasks somewhat more slowly, but with sufficient time, they are still able to accomplish them accurately.

After reaching approximately 60 years of age, there is a gradual decrease in the number of cells present in the spinal cord. However, this change typically does not have a significant impact on strength or sensation.

Digestive System

The aging process doesn't affect the digestive system as much as it affects other body parts. You can expect some minor changes, but they are so subtle that you might not even notice them. One of the minor noticeable changes, however, is a reduction in the forcefulness of muscle contractions in the esophagus, which is the tube that carries food from the throat to the stomach. It's a good thing this doesn't affect the movement of food through the esophagus itself.

Food will also begin to empty from the stomach at a slightly slower rate. Your stomach also becomes less elastic, meaning it cannot expand to hold as much food as before. Again, these are minor changes for most people, and therefore they won't cause any noticeable problems.

However, certain changes in the digestive system can lead to issues for some individuals. One example is a decrease in the production of lactose, an enzyme required to digest lactose, the sugar found in milk and dairy products. When the production of lactose decreases, people develop lactose intolerance. Older people with this condition may experience bloating, gas, or diarrhea after consuming dairy products. Additionally, the movement of materials through the large intestine tends to slow down with age, which can contribute to constipation in some people.

The liver also undergoes changes as a person ages. It tends to decrease in size due to a reduction in the number of liver cells. As a result, blood flow through the liver, and the efficiency of liver enzymes responsible for processing drugs and other substances in the body declines. Consequently, the liver may be somewhat less effective in removing drugs and substances from the body, causing the effects of these substances to last longer. This can have both intended and unintended consequences in terms of drug effects.

Overall, age-related changes in the digestive system are normally nothing to worry about. Most people won't experience any significant impact on the overall function of their system. With the exception of more uncomfortable and sometimes severe issues like lactose intolerance and constipation, you're more likely to maintain your overall health and function in this regard.

Heart and Blood Vessels

Our heart and blood vessels experience a loss of elasticity as we age. Generally, they become stiffer. This stiffness affects our ability to function optimally. Specifically, the heart fills with blood at a slower rate, and the arteries, which are responsible for carrying blood throughout the body, become less capable of expanding when there is a greater volume of blood to pump. This explains the increase in blood pressure in older adults.

Despite these age-related alterations, a healthy older heart generally functions adequately under normal conditions. The differences between young and old hearts become more evident when the heart is required to work harder, such as during physical exercise or periods of illness. An older heart is not as responsive in speeding up its rate or pumping as forcefully or efficiently as a younger heart. Have you ever wondered why older athletes are usually unable to perform as well as their younger counterparts? Now you have the answer.

However, with regular exercise, one can improve athletic performance regardless of age. And for those of us who aren't athletes, it can improve our overall well-being. Moreover, even the overall function and capabilities of the heart will benefit a great deal from an active lifestyle.

A sedentary lifestyle isn't an option at this point. With the exception of those battling complete immobility, we need to move around as much as we can. This is where the need for low-impact and gentle chair exercises is clearly portrayed.

Lungs and the Muscle of Breathing

The muscles involved in respiration, such as the diaphragm and intercostal muscles between the ribs, tend to experience a decline in strength. That's not all; even the number of air sacs (alveoli) and capillaries present in the lungs will begin to decrease. Overall, that will result in a slightly reduced absorption of oxygen from the inhaled air.

The lungs also experience a reduction in their elasticity. If you don't smoke or have a lung disorder, these changes generally won't disrupt your regular daily activities. However, they may contribute to increased difficulty during physical exercise. You can also expect breathing to become increasingly challenging at higher altitudes with lower oxygen levels.

Our lungs also become less effective at fighting infections, partially due to a decrease in the efficiency of the cells responsible for clearing debris and microorganisms from the airways. The strength of the cough reflex, which aids in clearing the lungs, also tends to diminish.

Ears

Most hearing changes, including hearing loss, can be traced back to a combination of long-term exposure to loud noise and the natural aging process. However, certain changes in hearing occur with age regardless of noise exposure. When hearing loss results from accumulated earwax, medical doctors can easily treat it.

Moreover, it's common for older adults to have a hard time hearing high-pitched sounds. Specialists call this age-related hearing loss or presbycusis. When you have this problem, even the clarity of violin music may be perceived as less pronounced.

With presbycusis comes a very frustrating predicament: the increased difficulty in understanding words. As a result, older adults may hear or perceive normal conversations as mumbling. Even when people speak louder, older individuals still struggle to comprehend the words. This difficulty arises because most consonant sounds (such as k, t, s, p, and ch) are high-pitched, and consonants play a crucial role in word identification. However, lower-pitched sound vowels are easier to hear.

Thus, older individuals may hear sentences like "Tell me exactly what you want to keep" as "Ell me exaly wha you wan oo ee." It is beneficial if people around them make an effort to enunciate consonants clearly instead of just speaking louder.

Understanding speech from women and children may pose more challenges compared to men because women and children generally have higher-pitched voices. However, older adults can also expect a gradual decline in their ability to hear lower-pitched sounds.

Endocrine System

The production and activity of certain hormones, which are synthesized by endocrine glands, decrease as we age. The following is more insight into this matter:

- The levels of growth hormone decrease, resulting in a decline in muscle mass.
- Aldosterone levels may significantly decrease, which increases the likelihood of dehydration. Aldosterone is responsible for signaling the body to retain salt and, consequently, water.
- The effectiveness of insulin, a hormone that regulates blood sugar (glucose) levels, diminishes. The production of insulin may decrease. Insulin facilitates the movement of sugar from the blood into cells, where it can be converted into energy. Consequently, when there are alterations in insulin levels, there will be a more pronounced increase in blood sugar levels following a large meal and a delayed return to normal levels.

While these changes may elevate the risk of health issues, they go unnoticed by most individuals. That is because these changes in the endocrine system hardly affect the overall health of older adults.

Moreover, while changes in insulin levels increase the likelihood of developing type 2 diabetes, regular exercise and a balanced diet plays a more crucial role in enhancing the action of insulin. I came to the conclusion that I'm not going to live in fear of these age-related challenges and health issues. Rather, I'm going to stay true to my exercise routine as I eat right so that I can give both my mental and physical health the best shot.

Eyes

Several changes also occur in vision as follows:

- The lens of the eye stiffens, making it more challenging to focus on objects up close.
- The lens becomes denser, resulting in difficulties seeing clearly in dim lighting conditions.
- The pupil reacts with slower responsiveness to changes in light.
- The lens gradually acquires a yellowish tint, altering the perception of colors.
- The decrease in the number of nerve cells affects depth perception, leading to a potential impairment.
- The eyes produce less fluid, causing a sensation of dryness.

It's common for a change in vision to serve as the initial undeniable indication of aging. Changes in the lenses of the eye can lead to or contribute to the following vision-related effects:

- **Loss of near vision:**

People often experience difficulty seeing objects closer than two feet as they reach their 40s. This condition is known as presbyopia, and it's a change that occurs when the eye's lens stiffens. Since the lens typically adjusts its shape to aid in focusing, a stiffened lens makes it harder to focus on nearby objects. This is how people develop presbyopia and start needing reading glasses with magnification. Those who already wear glasses for distance vision may need bifocals or lenses with variable focus.

- **Increased need for brighter light:**

With advancing age, seeing clearly in dim lighting becomes more challenging as the lens tends to lose transparency. A denser lens allows less light to pass through to the retina at the back of the eye. As if that's not enough, the retina, which contains light-sensing cells, becomes less sensitive. Brighter lighting becomes necessary for tasks like reading. On average, 60-year-olds require approximately three times more light for reading compared to 20-year-olds.

- **Changes in color perception:**

Color perception is also altered to some extent as the lens tends to develop a yellowish hue over time. Colors may appear less vibrant, making distinguishing contrasts between different colors a difficult task. While blues may appear grayer, blue text or backgrounds may appear faded. Although these changes are generally insignificant for most people, older people may find it harder to read black letters on a blue background or read blue-colored text.

- **Slower pupil reaction to light changes:**

The pupil of the eye expands and contracts to regulate the amount of light entering the eye based on the surrounding brightness. However, as we age, it begins to have a reduced reaction to our environment and the light it holds. As a result, seniors may find it harder to see in a dark room upon entry. They may even experience temporary blindness when entering a brightly lit area. Older individuals may also become more sensitive to glare. However, heightened sensitivity to glare is often associated with areas of darkness in the lens or the presence of cataracts.

Overall, subtle details like variations in shades and tones become harder to distinguish due to a decline in the number of nerve cells responsible for transmitting visual signals from the eyes to the brain. This is also why seniors may find it challenging to accurately judge distances.

Seniors may also start noticing an increase in the presence of tiny moving black specks in their field of vision. These specks are known as floaters and are solidified fragments of normal eye fluid. Floaters don't significantly impair vision or pose any health risks unless their frequency suddenly intensifies.

Additionally, seniors may experience dryness in their eyes as a result of a decrease in the production of fluids that lubricate the eyes. Overall, that change stems from a decline in the number of cells responsible for this function (producing fluids to lubricate the eyes). This may cause a notable reduction in tear production.

Changes In Appearance

The eyes undergo various changes in their appearance:

- The eyes may take on a subtle yellow or brown hue due to exposure to wind, ultraviolet light, and dust.
- Seniors with a darker complexion may notice sporadic patches of color on the whites of their eyes.
- A gray-white ring (arcus senilis) composed of calcium and cholesterol salts may start showing on the eye's surface. However, it has no impact on vision.
- Due to weakened eye muscles and stretched tendons, the lower eyelid may droop away from the eyeball. This condition, also known as ectropion, can impede proper eyeball lubrication and contribute to dry eyes.
- The eye may appear to recede into the head as the amount of fat surrounding the eye decreases.

Immune System

The immune system's cellular response becomes sluggish with age. Because these cells play an essential role in identifying and eliminating foreign substances like bacteria, other infectious agents, and potentially cancerous cells, their reduced efficiency has a negative impact on overall health. Let's take a look at some potential health hazards associated with reduced immune efficiency in older individuals:

- Increased risk of cancer.
- Reduced vaccine efficacy. However, vaccines for influenza, pneumonia, and shingles remain essential and provide some level of protection.
- Increased risk of infections like pneumonia and influenza. These infections may result in higher mortality rates.

Kidneys and Urinary Tract

Kidney size decreases due to a decline in the number of cells. As a result, there is reduced blood flow through the kidneys, which leads to a gradual decline in filtration capacity. This change is gradual and typically begins around the age of 30. With time, the kidneys may become less efficient at removing waste products from the blood, resulting in excessive water excretion and insufficient salt excretion. Overall, this increases the risk of dehydration. Nonetheless, the kidneys generally maintain sufficient functionality to meet the body's needs.

Moreover, age-related changes in the urinary tract can contribute to difficulties in controlling urination, including:

- decreased maximum bladder capacity, which causes more frequent urination in older individuals
- unpredictable contractions of the bladder muscles (overactive bladder), regardless of the need to urinate
- weakening of the bladder muscles, which results in incomplete bladder emptying and residual urine remaining after urination

- diminished ability of the urinary sphincter (muscle controlling urine passage) to close tightly, leading to difficulties in postponing urination and an increased likelihood of leakage

These changes contribute to the higher prevalence of urinary incontinence (uncontrolled loss of urine) as people age. In women, the urethra (the tube through which urine is expelled) tends to shorten, and its lining becomes thinner. Additionally, the decrease in estrogen levels during menopause may further contribute to these changes and cause other alterations in the urinary tract.

On the other hand, male individuals can expect their prostate glands to enlarge. In many cases, it enlarges sufficiently to obstruct urine flow and prevent complete emptying of the bladder. Consequently, older men may experience weaker urine flow, delayed initiation of urination, post-void dribbling, and increased frequency of urination. Older men also have a higher risk of urinary retention, the inability to urinate despite having a full bladder, requiring prompt medical attention.

Mouth and Nose

As people reach their 50s, they may begin to experience a gradual decline in their ability to taste and smell. This is an unwelcome change for any individual because both senses play a crucial role in fully appreciating the diverse flavors of food, and most of us love food! Moreover, the tongue can detect only five primary tastes: sweet, sour, bitter, salty, and umami (often described as savory or meaty). To discern more intricate and complex flavors like raspberry, the sense of smell is necessary.

As taste buds on the tongue become less sensitive, one's perception of sweetness and saltiness is affected. The sense of smell diminishes due to two reasons:

- a thinning and drying of the nasal lining
- the deterioration of nerve endings in the nose

However, these changes only have a subtle impact, and they primarily affect delicate aromas. This means that many foods may taste more bitter, while those with subtle scents may seem bland. Another notable change is how dryness in the mouth becomes more common as saliva production decreases. This dry mouth condition further impairs the ability to taste food.

As if that's not enough, gums may slightly recede, leading to exposure of the lower parts of the teeth to food particles and bacteria. Tooth enamel also tends to wear away. These changes, combined with a dry mouth, increase the susceptibility of teeth to decay and cavities, raising the likelihood of tooth loss.

Lastly, the nose may elongate, enlarge, and exhibit a drooping tip. That's not all; hairs in the nose, on the upper lip, and on the chin grow thicker.

Muscles and Fat

At age 30, going forward, people experience a gradual decline in muscle mass (muscle tissue) and muscle strength. This decline, unfortunately, persists throughout life. Several factors influence this change, including physical inactivity and declining levels of growth hormone and testosterone (both of which play a role in muscle development).

Moreover, there is a greater decline in fast-contracting (fast-twitch) muscle fibers compared to slow-contracting (slow-twitch) muscle fibers, leading to a decrease in the speed of muscle contraction. However, the impact of aging on muscle mass and strength is generally limited to a decrease of approximately 10–15% over the course of adulthood (Stefanacci, 2022).

With regular exercise, healthy seniors don't lose their muscle mass beyond 10–15%. It's important to note that more significant muscle loss, known as sarcopenia (meaning loss of flesh), is primarily caused by disease or extreme inactivity rather than aging.

In spite of these age-related changes, most seniors retain sufficient muscle mass and strength for daily activities. However, even the most physically fit individuals may experience some degree of decline as they age.

You can delay the loss of muscle mass and strength by engaging in regular muscle-strengthening exercises (muscle training). These exercises involve contracting muscles against resistance, which can be provided by gravity. Cardio and weight-bearing exercises are good examples, all of which can be achieved by low-impact chair exercises.

Through chair exercises, even those who have never exercised before can enhance their muscle mass and strength. On the other hand, prolonged physical inactivity can accelerate the loss of muscle mass and strength. Older individuals experience a faster decline in muscle mass and strength during periods of inactivity compared to younger individuals.

Lastly, as individuals reach 75 years of age, their body fat percentage generally doubles compared to their younger adult years. This increase in body fat also raises the risk of health issues such as diabetes. Furthermore, the distribution of fat throughout the body changes and alters the shape of the torso. To minimize these changes, seniors should adopt a healthy lifestyle by consuming a healthy diet and exercising regularly. What better way to achieve this than doing chair exercises in the comfort of your own home?

Reproductive Organs

When it comes to sex hormone levels, the impact of aging is more pronounced in women compared to men. In women, these effects are primarily associated with menopause, which comes with a notable decline in female hormones, particularly estrogen. Menopause marks the permanent cessation of menstrual periods and the end of the possibility of pregnancy.

When female hormone levels reduce, ovaries also shrink. Vaginal tissues also become thinner, drier, and less elastic (the term for this condition is atrophic vaginitis). These changes come with itching, bleeding, pain during intercourse, and urinary urgency when severe.

As if that's not enough, breast tissue becomes less firm and more fibrous, resulting in increased sagging. It becomes much more challenging to detect breast lumps at this stage of life.

Did You Know?

Age-related changes in breasts make it harder to identify any potential cancerous lumps.

Also, some of the changes that commence during menopause may negatively impact sexual activity (decreased hormone levels and vaginal dryness). However, for most women, aging doesn't significantly diminish the enjoyment of sexual activity. The absence of concerns regarding pregnancy can, in fact, enhance sexual activity and overall enjoyment.

Conversely, changes in sex hormone levels are more gradual in men than women. Additionally, the gradual decline in levels of the male hormone testosterone results in a decrease in sperm production and a lower sex drive (libido). However, this decline is not sudden because while there may be a reduction in blood flow to the penis, most men continue to experience erections and orgasms throughout their lives.

These erections, however, may not be as sustained as when men are younger, as they are slightly less firm and may often require more stimulation to maintain. It may also take longer for a second erection to occur. Erectile dysfunction (impotence) is more common in men as they age, resulting from disorders that affect blood vessels (vascular disease) or conditions like diabetes.

Skin

As individuals age, several changes occur in the skin. It gets thinner, less elastic, and drier. You will also notice that it will look finely wrinkled. However, prolonged exposure to sunlight over the years significantly contributes to wrinkling, roughness, and the development of blotchy skin. People who have actively avoided sunlight exposure often appear younger than their actual age.

These skin changes are partly attributed to chemical modifications and reduced flexibility of collagen (a tough, fibrous tissue that provides strength to the skin) and elastin (a protein that imparts skin with its flexibility). Moreover, the body's production of collagen and elastin significantly reduces with age, which explains why seniors are more prone to skin tearing.

The fat layer beneath the skin thins, diminishing its cushioning effect and protective support for the skin. This layer also aids in retaining body heat. With its thinning, people develop wrinkles and lose their tolerance for the cold.

As if that's not enough, there's a reduction in blood flow within deeper skin layers along with the number of sweat glands and blood vessels. Consequently, the body becomes less efficient at transferring heat from the inner body to the skin's surface through blood vessels. This impairs heat dissipation, making it more challenging for the body to cool itself effectively. This explains why seniors are more prone to heatstroke and other heat-related issues. Moreover, reduced blood flow slows down the skin's healing process.

The skin's protection against ultraviolet radiation isn't so strong at this point, as melanocytes decrease (pigment-producing cells). Consequently, large brown spots, commonly known as age spots, develop on areas of the skin that have been exposed to sunlight as the skin becomes less capable of effectively eliminating waste products.

The skin also becomes less efficient at synthesizing vitamin D upon exposure to sunlight, raising the risk of vitamin D deficiency.

COMMON ISSUES THAT MAY ARISE

There are common issues associated with getting older that you might not remember experiencing when you were younger. Suddenly, things that came naturally to you, like mobility, memory, and sleep, may become an everyday struggle. It's imperative that we discuss these issues, their early warning signs, why they happen, and how they can affect our lives. By gaining this perspective, we will know the importance of regular exercise and how it will positively change our lives.

Declined Mobility

When an elderly individual experiences a fall resulting in a hip fracture or develops a health condition such as Parkinson's disease, it becomes evident that they will face mobility challenges, even if those challenges are temporary. However, mobility difficulties are not solely caused by diseases or injuries. The natural aging process brings about factors like muscle loss, balance issues, and joint stiffness, all of which contribute to a decline in mobility.

Fortunately, older adults don't have to wait for an unfortunate incident to realize that they are encountering mobility issues.

There are certain warning signs that can indicate the potential or onset of mobility problems. By being observant and recognizing these signs, you can take proactive measures to enhance your balance and strength before any mishaps occur. This approach enables you to maintain your mobility and independence for as long as possible. Here are five crucial warning signs you should be mindful of regarding mobility (Hegg, n.d.):

- **Falling:**

Regardless of whether you appear to have resilient bones and seldom sustain serious injuries from falls, it's essential to address any underlying mobility issues before they worsen. Even experiencing just a couple of falls within a year may indicate a problem beyond environmental factors like uneven surfaces or cluttered surroundings. Falls can occur due to tripping over objects, dragging feet that struggle to keep up with movement, or losing balance and being unable to correct body positioning in time. Frequent falls significantly increase the risk of injuries, hospitalization, and potentially life-threatening complications. Therefore, it's highly recommended to take measures to make your living environment fall-proof by installing grab bars, handrails on stairs, non-slip tub mats, and other safety aids, even if you haven't yet sustained serious injuries. Additionally, it's important to consult your doctor and have your mobility evaluated. The doctor can assess any underlying health conditions that may be contributing to mobility problems, identify any adverse side effects of medications, or recommend physical therapy to enhance balance and strength.

- **Experiencing challenges when transitioning between sitting and standing:**

Do you struggle when attempting to rise from the couch? Are you finding it challenging to lower yourself into bed? Encountering difficulties with sitting and standing serves as a significant indication of potential mobility problems. These actions are fundamental in everyday life, such as when having meals, using the restroom, getting up in the morning or going to sleep, and more. Consider engaging in a quick and straight-forward sit-to-stand exercise and observe if you face any difficulties. Do you require support from furniture to maintain balance? Are you slow or unsteady in your movements? Recognizing such seemingly innocuous warning signs prompts the need to have a conversation with your doctor. Inquire about issues like lightheadedness or dizziness experienced during standing up or sitting down, and discuss the possibility of incorporating strength and balance exercises into your routine.

- **Opting to bypass the use of stairs:**

Do you frequently suggest taking the elevator when encountering even a small staircase while out and about? Have you caught yourself spending an extended amount of time downstairs in your home? You're not alone. For seniors, navigating stairs can be particularly challenging as it requires additional strength, balance, and energy. If you generally move around with relative ease but actively avoid using stairs, it may be worth discussing whether you require additional assistance or a mobility aid. If there are no apparent physical difficulties hindering your ability to navigate stairs, it's possible that a fear of falling is deterring you. Addressing these concerns and finding ways to alleviate yourself can have a positive impact on your long-term mobility.

- **Experiencing difficulties maintaining balance:**

Experiencing dizziness and encountering difficulties with balance can stem from various factors, including medication side effects, low blood pressure, or inner ear conditions such as vertigo or Meniere's disease. Furthermore, age-related issues such as impaired vision, joint stiffness, slower reaction times, and muscle weakness can compromise the body's ability to maintain balance, making activities like walking, standing, and exercising challenging. In order to enhance mobility, it is advisable for you to consult with your doctor for a balance assessment and treatment of any underlying issues. Incorporating mobility aids like canes or walkers, along with targeted exercises, can greatly assist with balance problems, enabling you to move around with increased safety and confidence.

- **Neglecting physical exercise:**

Engaging in regular exercise may not be everyone's preferred activity, but it is a vital habit for maintaining a healthy lifestyle and preventing chronic diseases, particularly for seniors. However, if you progressively skip exercise due to fatigue, soreness, or a lack of energy, you may soon encounter mobility issues. The weakness, exhaustion, and other symptoms that hinder your ability to exercise will gradually make it more challenging for you to walk or stand as extensively as you used to.

Common Causes

Limited mobility can manifest in different degrees, with individuals experiencing varying levels of challenges. For some, it may be difficult to walk long distances, while for others, it may result in complete immobility, rendering them unable to move their bodies. Below are some of the common causes associated with limited mobility in older adults (May, 2020):

Arthritis

Arthritis is a condition characterized by inflammation of the joints. It not only causes considerable pain but can also lead to joint degradation, resulting in stiffness and loss of functionality. Effective management of arthritis often involves a combination of medication and physical therapy. Therefore, if you're experiencing symptoms of stiff or painful joints, it's crucial to consult a doctor for appropriate guidance and treatment.

Osteoporosis

As we age, we experience a decline in bone density, which can result in weakened and brittle bones. Seniors diagnosed with osteoporosis often endure generalized bone pain, making movement uncomfortable. Additionally, they face an increased risk of fractures, further hindering their mobility. Fortunately, osteoporosis is often preventable. Adequate intake of calcium and vitamin D through a balanced diet is the primary means of avoiding this condition.

Heart Issues

Seniors who have coronary disease, heart failure, or other cardiac issues may experience difficulties with efficient oxygen circulation throughout their bodies. This can result in weakness and fatigue, making physical movement exhausting. Managing blood pressure and cholesterol levels can help seniors reduce their risk of heart problems.

Limited Balance and Coordination

Many seniors encounter diminished balance and coordination, leading them to limit their movements due to fear of falling. However, balance and coordination are skills that can be improved through practice. Physical therapy, exercise, and yoga are beneficial for strengthening the small muscles necessary for maintaining balance. Additionally, outfitting your home with handrails and other assistive devices can enhance your safety and mobility.

Reduced Hearing and Eyesight

Diminished vision and hearing can cause many seniors to experience a loss of mobility due to concerns about moving around safely. If you observe that your mobility is decreasing despite your overall health, it may be beneficial to consider scheduling hearing and vision tests. By addressing these sensory impairments with the use of glasses, hearing aids, or other appropriate treatments, it's possible to restore confidence and enhance mobility, enabling you to move around more comfortably and securely.

Obesity

Obesity poses a greater concern for older individuals compared to other age groups. This is due to the increased pressure it places on the musculoskeletal system, resulting in pain and stress that negatively impact mobility. Additionally, obesity can contribute to the development of conditions such as osteoarthritis and diabetes, further diminishing mobility.

To enhance your quality of life, you should strive to increase physical activity and make dietary adjustments, including incorporating more vegetables, fruits, and fish into your meals.

Increased Pain

Chronic pain is becoming more prevalent among older patients, mainly caused by conditions such as arthritis, cancer, diabetes mellitus, and cardiovascular and neurologic diseases. Furthermore, as we adopt a holistic approach to pain management that considers the biopsychosocial aspects, it becomes crucial to examine how lifestyle changes associated with aging can contribute to the worsening of pain syndromes.

Older patients often take multiple medications for their various medical conditions, which increases the risk of side effects and even mortality related to these drugs. Additionally, it's important to understand and address certain dynamics of pharmacotherapy when making decisions about medication management. These dynamics encompass the following (Robeck, 2012):

- As individuals age, they experience a greater proportion of body fat and a decline in body water and muscle mass. Consequently, water-soluble drugs become more concentrated and have higher initial concentrations in older adults. On the other hand, fat-soluble drugs have extended half-lives because they are released more slowly from the body's fat reserves.
- As people age, the liver tends to shrink in size and receive less blood flow, resulting in a decrease in the number of working liver cells. Additionally, medications can affect the liver's ability to process drugs. These changes in liver function and drug metabolism emphasize the importance of personalized considerations when prescribing medications to older patients.
- The rise in renal disease prevalence has significant implications for medication choices affected by renal clearance or known to elevate the risk of renal damage. Even in the absence of diagnosed renal disease, older patients often experience a notable decline in renal clearance, which can influence the adverse event profile of several medications that are generally well-tolerated by younger patients.

Treating chronic pain in older individuals can be complex, but the benefits of addressing and managing pain are evident. Chronic pain not only diminishes functionality but also raises the risk of depression, fosters kinesiophobia (fear of movement), and can exacerbate other chronic diseases that require ongoing management, such as diabetes, hypertension, and heart disease.

Pain hampers patients' ability to concentrate, sleep, and cope with everyday stressors, ultimately diminishing their overall quality of life. Inadequately managed pain not only compromises patients' well-being but also significantly increases healthcare costs. Unfortunately, the pursuit of quick and affordable pain relief has often resulted in potentially hazardous polypharmacy, neglecting nonpharmacologic options.

Increased Risk of Falls

Falls have become a significant public health concern, especially among the aging population in the United States. They stand as the leading cause of injury and injury-related deaths for older adults (aged 65+), with an unfortunate occurrence of a fall every second of every day. Shockingly, one in four older adults experiences a fall each year in the United States (Centers for Disease Control and Prevention [CDC], 2023).

Why Is There an Increase in Falls as People Age?

Extensive research has identified numerous risk factors that play a role in falls, and it has been determined that some of these factors are modifiable. The majority of falls occur due to the interplay of multiple risk factors. As the number of risk factors increases, so does the likelihood of a person experiencing a fall. Healthcare providers have the ability to decrease an individual's risk by addressing and mitigating their specific risk factors, thus reducing the chances of falling (CDC, 2017).

In order to prevent falls, you can consult with your healthcare providers and communicate your health goals with them. By doing so, they can identify the modifiable fall risk factors that can be targeted to assist you in achieving your goals. Subsequent chapters will teach you low-impact chair exercises to help with posture, build strength, and more. These exercises will help to prevent falls. It's also wise to mention them to your healthcare provider on your next visit.

Moreover, there are effective clinical and community interventions available for various fall risk factors, including:

- vestibular dysfunction or poor balance
- inadequate levels of vitamin D
- medications that are associated with falls
- postural hypotension (low blood pressure upon standing)
- impaired vision
- foot or ankle disorders
- hazards within the home environment

By addressing these specific risk factors, healthcare providers can implement appropriate interventions to reduce the likelihood of falls and promote your safety.

Did You Know?

Based on findings from the U.S. Centers for Disease Control and Prevention (CDC) and other studies on falls (National

Council on Aging, 2023):

- More than 25% of Americans aged 65 and above experience falls each year.
- Falls are the primary cause of fatal and nonfatal injuries among older adults.
- The projected cost of treating fall-related injuries is expected to surpass $101 billion by 2030.
- Falls lead to over 3 million injuries treated in emergency departments annually, including more than 800,000 hospitalizations.
- In 2015, the total expenses related to nonfatal fall injuries reached $50 billion.
- Medical costs associated with fatal falls amount to approximately $754 million each year.
- Fall death rates for older adults in the United States increased by 30% from 2007 to 2016, with a projected estimation of 7 deadly falls per hour by 2030.
- Individuals with mild hearing loss are nearly three times more likely to experience falls, with every 10 decibels of hearing loss increasing the risk.
- Approximately 60% of falls occur at home, while 30% take place in public settings, and 10% happen in healthcare centers.

OTHER COMMON ISSUES

I'm a firm believer that when we familiarize ourselves with these prevalent chronic conditions, we can proactively take measures to prevent disease and maintain our well-being as we grow older. Let's take a look at most health issues we need to watch out for and combat (Vann, 2016):

Arthritis

Arthritis affects a significant portion of individuals aged 65 and older. While arthritis can potentially discourage physical activity, it's crucial to collaborate with your doctor to develop a personalized activity plan that, when combined with appropriate treatment, can contribute to the maintenance of senior health.

Heart Disease

As reported by the CDC, heart disease continues to be the leading cause of death among adults aged 65 and above. According to the Federal Interagency Forum on Aging-Related Statistics, this chronic condition affects 37% of men and 26% of women in this age group (Vann, 2016). As individuals age, they become more susceptible to risk factors like high blood pressure and high cholesterol, which elevate the likelihood of experiencing a stroke or developing heart disease. To address this health risk among seniors, Dr. Bernard recommends a holistic approach that not only aids in managing heart disease but also enhances overall senior health (Vann, 2016): "Engage in regular exercise, maintain a healthy and well-balanced diet to achieve and maintain a healthy weight, and prioritize adequate sleep for optimal well-being."

Cancer

According to the CDC, cancer ranks as the second leading cause of death for individuals aged 65 and above. The CDC states that 28% of men and 21% of women in this age group live with cancer (Vann, 2016). Early detection through screenings like mammograms, colonoscopies, and skin checks can significantly increase the treatability of many types of cancer. While preventing cancer is not always possible, seniors living with cancer can enhance their quality of life, including during treatment, by collaborating with their medical team and adhering to healthy senior living recommendations.

Respiratory Disease

Seniors with chronic respiratory diseases face increased health risks, making them more susceptible to infections like pneumonia. However, preserving senior health and maintaining a satisfactory quality of life can be achieved by undergoing lung function tests, adhering to the correct medication, and following prescribed oxygen therapy guidelines.

Alzheimer's Disease

Alzheimer's disease, as per the CDC, resulted in 92,604 deaths among individuals aged 65 and above in 2014. Moreover, the Alzheimer's Association states that approximately 11% (or one in nine) of people in this age group are affected by Alzheimer's disease (Vann, 2016). However, due to the complexity of the diagnosis, the exact number of individuals living with this chronic condition is challenging to ascertain. Nevertheless, experts acknowledge that cognitive impairment significantly impacts senior health in various aspects, ranging from safety and self-care to the financial burden of caregiving, whether provided at home or in a residential facility.

Osteoporosis

According to Dr. Bernard, osteoporosis can lead to reduced mobility and potential disability, particularly if a fall results in fractures or vertebral body collapse (Vann, 2016). The National Osteoporosis Foundation reports that approximately 54 million Americans aged 50 and above are affected by low bone mass or osteoporosis, making them vulnerable to fractures that can negatively impact senior health and diminish the quality of life (Vann, 2016).

Diabetes

Around 25% of individuals aged 65 and older are affected by diabetes, which poses a substantial health risk for seniors, as estimated by the CDC (Vann, 2016). In 2014 alone, diabetes accounted for 54,161 deaths among adults in this age group, according to CDC data. Early detection and management of diabetes are possible through simple blood tests to measure blood sugar levels. Being aware of your diabetes status or risk enables you to make timely lifestyle changes to control the disease and enhance your long-term outlook for senior health (Vann, 2016).

Influenza and Pneumonia

While not chronic conditions, the flu and pneumonia rank among the top eight causes of death in individuals aged 65 and above, as outlined by the CDC (Vann, 2016). Seniors are particularly susceptible to these infections and may have a weakened ability to combat them. In order to prevent these diseases and their potentially life-threatening complications, it is recommended that seniors receive an annual flu shot and, if advised by their healthcare provider, the pneumonia vaccine. Following these senior healthcare recommendations can help safeguard against these infections and protect overall well-being.

Obesity

Obesity represents a significant senior health risk factor, contributing to conditions such as heart disease, diabetes, and cancer, all of which can have a considerable impact on quality of life. As body weight increases, so does the risk of developing these diseases. According to the CDC, 36.2% of men and 40.7% of women aged 65 to 74 fall into the obese category, indicated by a body mass index (BMI) equal to or greater than 30 (Vann, 2016). Additionally, obesity can serve as a signal that older adults may not be as physically active or mobile as they once were.

Depression

According to the American Psychological Association, approximately 15–20% of Americans aged 65 and above have encountered depression (Vann, 2016). This poses a threat to senior health as depression can weaken the immune system and hinder the ability to combat infections effectively. Alongside medication and therapy, there are other methods to enhance senior living. For instance, increasing physical activity could be beneficial, considering that 59.4% of adults aged 65 and older do not meet the exercise recommendations outlined by the CDC (Vann, 2016). Additionally, fostering more social interactions is advantageous. According to the Federal Interagency Forum on Aging-Related Statistics, seniors report spending only 8–11% of their free time with family and friends (Vann, 2016).

Muscle Strength

After reaching 40, muscle mass and strength begin to decline. By the time individuals reach the age of 85, around 20% of them meet the criteria for sarcopenia, which signifies a significant loss of muscle mass and strength (Jaul & Barron, 2017). Several factors likely contribute to sarcopenia, including chronic inflammation, decreasing hormone levels, impaired muscle mitochondrial function, and impaired muscle stem cell function.

This decline in muscle mass and the corresponding increase in fat mass have implications for pharmacokinetics, as older adults may require lower medication doses compared to younger adults. It is worth noting that muscle weakness and a rapid decline in strength are both indicators of future mortality.

EXERCISES CAN HELP

There's no better time to start making better health choices than now. If you've been thinking it's too late to start exercising, this is your cue to change your mind and start changing your life for the better, one simple chair exercise at a time. I'm rooting for you!

You Can Still Exercise With Limited Mobility

If you have limited mobility, gentle chair exercises will help you to exercise without having to move around a lot. Unfortunately, our bodies don't reward a sedentary lifestyle regardless of our health conditions. We need to stay as active as we can, and the good news is that there are suitable exercises for each stage of life.

Exercise can be safely enjoyed by the majority of adults over the age of 65, including those with chronic conditions and limited mobility. However, it is essential to consult with your doctor before embarking on any exercise program to determine the most suitable options based on your health and activity level. By taking this important step, you can confidently embrace the immense benefits of exercise and witness its positive impact on your overall well-being.

The Importance of Exercise

We have learned a lot about the health challenges associated with aging, but now it's time to delve into the benefits of exercise. All hope is not lost, and we all stand a chance to lead healthier and more fulfilling lives if we choose to eat right and maintain an active lifestyle. Here are some of the benefits of regular exercise for seniors (The National Council on Aging, 2021):

Prevents Bone Loss

As individuals age, both men and women experience a decline in bone density, with post-menopausal women facing a potential loss of up to 2% each year. However, research has demonstrated that strength training can effectively counteract this bone loss and even restore bone density. By engaging in regular strength training exercises, seniors can develop stronger bones, resulting in a reduced risk of fractures. Additionally, improved bone density can contribute to better balance, further lowering the risk of falls and injuries. By incorporating exercise into their routines, seniors can enhance their independence and enjoy an extended period of independent living.

Alleviates Discomfort from Osteoarthritis

Contrary to intuition, increasing physical activity can actually help alleviate the pain and stiffness associated with arthritis. Arthritis-friendly exercises encompass low-impact cardiovascular activities, strength training, and range-of-motion exercises. Exercise benefits arthritis by strengthening the muscles surrounding the affected joints by alleviating pressure on them. Physical activity may also assist in reducing joint inflammation and promoting lubrication, resulting in reduced pain and stiffness.

Aids in Chronic Disease Prevention

Engaging in regular exercise can protect you against chronic illnesses such as cardiovascular disease, colon cancer, diabetes, obesity, and hypertension. In cases where individuals already have a chronic condition, engaging in physical activity can help minimize symptoms and improve overall well-being. Furthermore, exercise has been shown to have potential benefits in reducing cognitive decline. A study revealed that individuals over the age of 60 who engaged in 30 minutes of exercise daily exhibited fewer Alzheimer's disease biomarkers (National Council on Aging, 2021). This highlights the positive impact of exercise on cognitive health in older adults.

Boosts Immunity

According to a study conducted in 2018, moderate exercise was associated with a reduced risk of acute respiratory illness and fewer missed work days due to sickness (National Council on Aging, 2021). While the exact mechanisms by which exercise supports the immune system are not fully understood, several theories have been proposed. One theory suggests that the anti-inflammatory effects of physical activity contribute to improved immune function. Additionally, exercise may enhance the performance of immune cells, further bolstering the body's defenses against illnesses.

Enhances Mood

In essence, exercise has a positive impact on our emotional well-being. It has the potential to alleviate symptoms of anxiety and depression, promote relaxation, and generate an overall sense of well-being. A study conducted in 2019 focusing on adult men aged 65 and older revealed that the mood-enhancing benefits of exercise persist well into old age (National Council on Aging, 2021). This emphasizes the crucial role of staying physically active in maintaining mental and emotional health throughout the aging process.

Promotes Sleep

Individuals with sedentary lifestyles often experience difficulties in obtaining restful sleep, but adopting an active lifestyle can aid in achieving better sleep. Incorporating regular aerobic exercise during the day promotes deeper sleep by increasing core body temperature and facilitating rest as the body cools down. Engaging in physical activity two to three hours before bedtime can help ensure a more sustained and refreshing sleep, allowing you to wake up feeling rejuvenated.

Builds Social Wellness

Maintaining an active social life can pose challenges for many seniors. However, some older adults are finding ways to enhance their social well-being by incorporating exercise into enjoyable group activities within their communities. From joining a walking group to participating in an aerobics class, combining socialization with physical activity can help you stay youthful at heart and mentally sharp. Engaging in exercise as a social outing allows seniors to foster connections, enjoy companionship, and experience the numerous benefits of both physical and social wellness.

How Much Exercise Should Seniors Get?

The amount of exercise recommended for seniors over 65 depends on their overall health, fitness level, and any underlying medical conditions. In general, 150 minutes of aerobic activity (moderate intensity) should suffice. You can divide this into 30-minute exercises during the week. Try to incorporate strength training exercises at least twice a week, targeting major muscle groups.

You can also engage in at least two to three hours of chair exercises each week, spread out over several sessions. This duration allows for a sufficient amount of physical activity to benefit cardiovascular health, muscle strength, flexibility, and balance. However, it's important to note that the duration may vary depending on individual abilities and health conditions.

You can also incorporate more activity into your day as follows:

- Go up the stairs and leave the elevator.
- Choose to walk or bike instead of driving for short distances.
- Take your dog for a walk.
- Engage in yard work or gardening.
- Perform light exercises while watching TV.

By incorporating these activities into your daily routine, you can enhance your overall physical fitness and well-being.

AGE IS JUST A NUMBER

A lady aged 103 continues to defy expectations and excel in sprinting. Besides winning gold medals in the 50 and 100-meter races in New Mexico, Julia "Hurricane" Hawkins set a new U.S.A. track and field record as the oldest woman to compete on an American track.

Hawkins, who began her running career at the age of 100, has a history of breaking records. She managed to establish three world records by age 102, including one in the 100-meter dash. Her determination and drive to compete at her age inspire others, and she hopes to encourage people to realize that they can continue pursuing their passions regardless of their age.

While gardening serves as her training secret, Hawkins also competes to impress her family. With her remarkable achievements and an ever-growing list of records, she is bound to inspire and impress many more individuals beyond her immediate circle (Dubois, 2019).

2

WHY CHAIR EXERCISES?

> *Exercise not only changes your body, it changes your mind, your attitude and your mood.*

— UNKNOWN

Physical fitness remains just as crucial for older individuals as it is for the younger population. We must maintain a certain level of fitness as we grow older. However, as we grow older, it may become challenging to engage in movements that strain our bodies or maintain balance. This is where chair exercises become valuable, particularly for those with limited mobility or difficulty maintaining balance.

Incorporating chair exercises into your daily routine helps decrease the risk of falls. These movements stimulate blood flow, keeping your joints active and well-lubricated. Additionally, chair exercises contribute to the strengthening of your muscles, promoting overall physical well-being. By consistently performing chair exercises, you can enjoy improved mobility, reduced fall risk, and enhanced muscular strength.

It's also common to spend more time in a seated position, which can have a negative impact on our posture. Regardless of age, it's essential to maintain good posture. When we sit, the pelvis tends to tilt backward, causing the bottom to tilt under. This can result in inadequate support for the upper half of our body from the hips. Moreover, sitting fails to engage the glutes and core muscles, which play a vital role in supporting the spine.

Over time, this can cause the spine to adopt a long C-curve shape instead of its natural S shape. This postural slump can gradually impair our ability to maintain an upright posture when standing. However, incorporating chair exercises into our routine can help prevent further deterioration of the situation.

Chair exercises target the muscles involved in maintaining good posture, such as the core and glutes. By regularly engaging in these exercises, we can strengthen these muscles, support the spine, and prevent the progression of poor posture. Ultimately, chair exercises play a crucial role in preserving and improving our posture as we age.

THE BENEFITS OF CHAIR EXERCISES

Not only are they convenient, but chair exercises have numerous benefits. Let's take a look:

Improved Posture

As we age, our ability to move and be independent often becomes increasingly limited. In highly congested areas, going for a short walk can be challenging, especially for those who no longer drive. Unfortunately, this loss of freedom frequently leads to reduced mobility and more sedentary lifestyles.

The longer you spend sitting, the more your joints tend to stiffen, potentially resulting in a permanent shift in posture that brings muscle pain and fatigue over time. As your posture deteriorates, the muscles in your lower body weaken, making it harder to support the upper half of your body. Prolonged sitting can also lead to weakened glutes and core muscles, which are crucial for supporting the spine.

To address these issues and enhance your core strength and posture, consider incorporating chair exercises into your routine, even during extended periods of sitting. Subsequent chapters will teach you more about them.

Increased Coordination

As we grow older, coordination can pose challenges, particularly for seniors diagnosed with conditions such as Alzheimer's, which affect cognitive abilities. However, engaging in repetitive exercises can assist in developing muscle memory, which can contribute to the retention of hand-eye coordination and promote greater independence.

Chair exercises not only enhance coordination but also contribute to joint health. Additionally, when performed in a group setting, they offer a valuable socializing experience for participants.

Reduced Pain

Engaging in exercise to improve senior mobility not only has the potential to reduce pain but also offers various other benefits. Physical exercise triggers the release of endorphins, which aid in reducing inflammation. Additionally, increased movement helps to lubricate the joints, minimizing discomfort associated with their use. Strengthening the core muscles also helps relieve strain on muscles, leading to reduced shoulder and back pain.

In general, the more you move, the less pain you are likely to experience. Our bodies are not designed to remain sedentary for extended periods. However, it's important to consider individual circumstances. If you are recovering from surgery or have a muscular or joint condition, it is advisable to consult your doctor regarding your exercise routine. Always follow the guidance provided by your doctor or physical therapist regarding the appropriate level of activity for your specific situation.

While all chair exercises can provide relief for certain types of pain, stretching and flexibility exercises like chair yoga are particularly effective. You can try stretching your arms overhead or in front of you, twisting your body gently, or reaching for the floor.

When performing a range of motion exercises, it is important to prioritize comfort and avoid pushing yourself to the point of actual pain. Excessive strain on your joints or muscles could result in damage.

Decreased Obesity

Low-impact chair exercises can effectively contribute to reducing obesity in seniors by providing a safe and accessible means of physical activity. By engaging in low-impact movements, seniors can burn calories and increase their metabolic rate. This calorie expenditure, coupled with a balanced diet, creates a calorie deficit necessary for weight loss.

Additionally, chair exercises improve cardiovascular health by elevating heart rate and promoting better circulation. Strengthening exercises targeting different muscle groups, including the arms, legs, and core, help seniors build muscle mass, which in turn increases metabolic rate. Chair exercises also enhance joint flexibility and mobility, reducing stiffness and improving physical function. By engaging in regular physical activity, seniors can boost their energy levels, reduce sedentary behavior, and improve overall well-being. Combined with psychological benefits such as improved mood and reduced stress, low-impact chair exercises offer a holistic approach to reducing obesity and promoting healthier lifestyles in seniors.

Decreased Bone Loss

Chair exercises can help reduce bone loss in seniors by providing weight-bearing activities that stimulate bone growth. When seniors engage in these exercises, such as knee lifts or chair running, they put stress on their bones, which triggers the bone-building process. This helps increase bone density and strength, reducing the risk of fractures and osteoporosis. Regular participation in chair exercises also improves muscle strength, balance, and coordination, which further protects against falls and bone injuries. By incorporating these exercises into your routine, you can maintain and enhance your bone health, promoting better overall skeletal strength and reducing the effects of age-related bone loss.

Disease Prevention

Low-impact chair exercises can help prevent diseases in seniors by promoting overall health and well-being. Regular participation in these exercises, such as chair running/marching or arm circles, improves cardiovascular fitness, reducing the risk of heart disease and high blood pressure. These exercises also help maintain a healthy weight, which lowers the chances of developing obesity-related conditions like diabetes.

Additionally, chair exercises enhance muscle strength and flexibility, improving mobility and reducing the risk of falls and injuries. By boosting the immune system, reducing stress, and enhancing mental health, these exercises contribute to a stronger immune response and a decreased risk of certain illnesses. Overall, low-impact chair exercises support seniors in maintaining a healthier lifestyle and reducing the likelihood of various diseases.

Reduced Risk of Falling

Chair exercises reduce the risk of falling in older adults. As individuals age, balance, strength, and flexibility tend to decline, making them more vulnerable to falls and related injuries. However, engaging in regular chair exercises can help mitigate these risks and improve overall stability and mobility.

Because chair exercises are specifically designed to be performed while seated, they are accessible and safe for older adults with limited mobility or balance issues. These exercises target various muscle groups, including the legs, core, and upper body, which play a crucial role in maintaining stability and preventing falls.

When you incorporate chair exercises into your daily routine, you significantly improve your strength, flexibility, and coordination. Stronger muscles, particularly in the lower body, provide better support and stability while walking or performing daily activities. Enhanced flexibility increases joint mobility and range of motion, reducing the likelihood of falls due to stiffness or limited movement.

Furthermore, chair exercises often focus on balance and posture, which are essential for maintaining stability. Through exercises that target balance, such as leg lifts or leg kicks, older adults can improve their proprioception (awareness of body position in space) and develop better control over their movements.

Regular participation in chair exercises also has positive effects on bone health. Weight-bearing exercises, even when performed while seated, help strengthen bones and reduce the risk of osteoporosis and fractures.

Moreover, chair exercises contribute to overall well-being and confidence in older adults. As they become stronger and more capable, individuals gain a sense of empowerment and independence, which can significantly boost self-esteem and reduce the fear of falling.

It is important to note that older adults should consult with a healthcare professional or a certified fitness instructor experienced in working with seniors before starting any exercise program. They can provide guidance on suitable chair exercises and help tailor a routine that addresses individual needs and limitations.

In conclusion, chair exercises offer a safe and effective way for older adults to reduce the risk of falling. By improving strength, flexibility, balance, and overall stability, these exercises promote independence, enhance well-being, and contribute to a healthier and more active lifestyle for older adults.

SETTING FITNESS GOALS

Embarking on a lifestyle change can be difficult, but setting goals can make it easier. Goals provide motivation, focus, and a way to track progress. When aiming to increase physical activity, it's important to set realistic and well-planned goals to stay on track and stay motivated. Before starting any exercise program, especially if you're over 40, overweight, have been inactive for a while, or have a chronic medical condition, it's crucial to go through a pre-exercise self-screening tool. This tool helps ensure your safety and provides valuable information to guide your physical activity journey. By setting achievable goals and taking necessary precautions, you can enhance your chances of success and enjoy the benefits of a more active lifestyle.

Key principles for setting physical activity goals include the following (Better Health Channel, n.d.-b):

- Identify your ultimate goal.
- Determine the steps to achieve your ultimate goal.
- Establish small and specific mini-goals.
- Regularly track and monitor your progress.
- Be flexible and adapt to changing circumstances.
- Practice self-compassion and avoid being too hard on yourself.

Common Fitness Goals

Individuals have diverse motivations and goals when it comes to exercise. Our bodies, fitness aspirations, and approaches vary. Consequently, many individuals opt to enlist the assistance of a personal trainer to support them in achieving their desired outcomes. Despite our differences, certain fitness goals frequently emerge, shared by numerous individuals or showing similarities. Let's explore some of these common fitness aims:

- **Fat loss:** Many individuals embark on an exercise journey to shed excess fat. In addition to regular workouts, seeking guidance on modifying eating habits, reducing caloric intake, and limiting carbohydrates are essential for achieving this goal.

- **Muscle building:** Some people aim to build muscle mass to improve their appearance and overall well-being. This goal involves challenging weightlifting sessions, extended workout durations, and increased protein intake. Consulting a personal trainer is recommended for effective muscle-building strategies.

- **Endurance improvement:** Individuals who easily get out of breath (after climbing a few flights of stairs, for example) are motivated to enhance their endurance. High-intensity interval training (HIIT) for 20 to 30 minutes, incorporating equipment like steppers or rowers, can be effective. The goal is to elevate the heart rate and consistently challenge oneself.

- **Flexibility enhancement:** Seeking professional guidance from a personal trainer is crucial for improving flexibility. They can evaluate your current flexibility level and provide appropriate exercises. Additionally, performing proprioceptive neuromuscular facilitation (PNF) and static stretches can be beneficial as long as they are done within safe limits and without pushing through pain.

- **Body toning:** Some individuals desire a toned physique without excessive muscle bulk or significant fat reduction. This goal requires a combination of exercise and dietary modifications. While toning may seem less challenging than building muscle, it still requires dedication and effort.

Regardless of your specific fitness goal, wearing appropriate workout attire that allows freedom of movement and promotes breathability is important for a comfortable and productive workout.

How to Design Your Personal Fitness Goals

Designing fitness goals is one thing, but sticking to them and remaining consistent is another. Overall, it takes skill to design fitness goals that can yield results, and the following are some well-researched tips just for you (McCoy 2019):

Concentrate on One Fitness Goal at a Time

Avoid trying to accomplish too much all at once. Instead of overwhelming yourself with multiple objectives simultaneously, it's important to focus on one goal at a time. Scantlebury, a certified strength and conditioning specialist and the founder of Fit Club NY, explains that attempting to tackle numerous goals simultaneously sets you up for failure (McCoy 2019). With an extensive list of tasks to accomplish, people often feel anxious and perceive themselves as failures if they fall short in any aspect. This negative self-talk can hinder your chances of achieving any of the goals.

Instead, it's recommended to choose a single objective to prioritize and direct your efforts toward its accomplishment. For instance, you might focus on mastering a pull-up or completing your first-ever 5K race. By concentrating on one goal at a time, you increase your likelihood of success before moving on to pursue another goal.

Own the Process

It's easy to become envious when scrolling through fitness-focused content on social media. However, it's wiser to avoid setting your own goals based on what others have achieved, as this approach is neither productive nor practical.

In today's world, we are constantly exposed to images and messages that dictate what fitness should look like and how we should go about achieving it. This barrage of information can make it challenging to discern what truly benefits us personally. Vidal, an NYC-based certified strength and conditioning specialist and master trainer with the fitness app POPiN, emphasizes that while certain accomplishments, such as running a marathon, doing 100 push-ups, or mastering complex yoga poses, may be impressive for top athletes, they shouldn't be the universal metrics by which everyone is measured (McCoy, 2019).

In essence, Vidal suggests that your goals should be tailored to you and your unique aspirations. They should be something that genuinely excites you and is realistically attainable rather than attempting to replicate someone else's achievements. By focusing on your own goals, you can maintain motivation and pursue a path that aligns with your individual capabilities and desires.

Set Specific, Measurable, Attainable, Relevant and Time-Bound Fitness Goals (SMART)

According to Vidal and the NYC-based certified strength and conditioning specialist DiSalvo, setting a measurable goal is crucial for tracking progress and achieving success (McCoy 2019). They emphasize that the more specific the goal, the clearer the path to attainment becomes. While having a general desire to "be stronger" is a good starting point, it's essential to define what that means to you personally. For instance, stating that you want to increase the number of push-ups you can do makes the goal measurable, and specifying that you aim to reach 20 push-ups in one minute makes it even more specific. Additionally, setting a timeframe for the goal creates a sense of urgency, focuses your efforts, and allows you to develop a structured plan for achievement.

The SMART method can help ensure your goals meet these criteria. By following this approach, you can establish goals that are specific to your needs, can be tracked and measured, are realistically attainable, hold relevance to your aspirations, and are bound by a specific timeframe. Using this method will increase your chances of successful goal attainment.

Start Small

According to Mike Clancy, a certified strength and conditioning specialist based in NYC, it's important for your goal to be attainable and seem relatively easy or within reach based on your current capabilities (McCoy, 2019). This is because perceiving your goal as easy indicates that you have already overcome any mental obstacles that could hinder your progress. Clancy explains that having a high level of confidence is crucial, ideally at a 9 out of 10, in terms of believing that you can truly achieve your goal. The more confident you are, the more likely you are to stick to the necessary steps to make it happen.

Setting attainable goals also has the advantage of providing early wins in your fitness journey. As Scantlebury points out, the more success you experience early on, the more motivated you will be to continue (McCoy, 2019). These initial victories build confidence, creating a positive momentum that can lead to long-term results. By starting with achievable goals, you set yourself up for success, fostering a sense of accomplishment that fuels your commitment to ongoing fitness pursuits.

Practice Patience

According to DiSalvo, it's crucial to be realistic when establishing the time frame for achieving your goal, despite the desire for instant gratification (McCoy, 2019). Lasting changes, he explains, take time and cannot be achieved overnight.

Scantlebury further emphasizes that expecting a complete overhaul in just one week is unrealistic. Instead, it's advisable to choose a goal that can be accomplished over the course of several months or even a year. Adopting a long-term mindset allows you to view your goal as a lifestyle change rather than a quick fix. This shift in perspective increases the likelihood of sticking to your goal and making sustainable progress. Understanding that meaningful transformations require time and dedication enables you to approach your fitness journey with patience and commitment, setting the stage for long-term success.

Know What Drives You

Occasionally, fitness goals can stem from deep-rooted fears, insecurities, or body image concerns; for instance, wanting to run a marathon due to past experiences of bullying in middle school gym class or enrolling in a CrossFit class because of a hurtful comment about weight from an ex-partner. It's crucial to recognize and address these underlying issues instead of assuming that achieving the fitness goal will automatically alleviate them.

According to DiSalvo, the pursuit of certain goals can evoke intense emotions (McCoy, 2019). If thoughts about your goal trigger anxiety or resurface past mental struggles, it is advisable to seek support from a mental health professional. They can provide valuable guidance and help you navigate the complex emotions associated with your fitness journey. By addressing these underlying concerns, you can develop a more holistic approach to your well-being, ensuring that both your physical and mental health are prioritized throughout the process.

Embrace Different Kinds of Success

While setting specific goals is important, it's equally crucial to give yourself the flexibility to modify them as you progress in your fitness journey. Sometimes, a goal that initially seemed appropriately challenging may turn out to be too difficult to sustain, or conversely, it might become too easy. According to

Vidal, if your definition of success is rigid and unyielding, it can be challenging to maintain motivation (McCoy, 2019).

Always set goals that are attainable, then gradually adjust them as you gain a better understanding of your capabilities. It is perfectly acceptable to move the goalposts as you become more acquainted with your body's abilities and limitations. Being open to modifying your goals allows for a more realistic and adaptable approach to your fitness journey. It ensures that your goals align with your evolving needs and empowers you to make adjustments that support continued progress and personal growth.

Set Small Goals as You Make Your Way to Bigger Ones

As part of your overarching goal, it's beneficial to incorporate smaller confidence-building goals that can be achieved within a shorter time frame. For instance, if your ultimate goal is to run a nine-minute mile, it is advisable to establish smaller milestones along the way. Setting a goal, like running a half mile in five minutes, allows you to gauge your progress and acknowledge your accomplishments. DiSalvo explains that celebrating these little victories is crucial for maintaining motivation and rewarding yourself mentally. Waiting too long to feel a sense of achievement can dampen your motivation and potentially derail your progress.

In general, Clancy suggests setting micro-goals that can be achieved every two to three weeks (McCoy, 2019). This time frame provides an opportunity to assess the realism of your larger goal and make necessary adjustments if needed. It serves as a valuable checkpoint to evaluate your progress, ensuring that your macro goal remains attainable. By breaking down your larger goal into smaller, achievable milestones and regularly evaluating your progress, you can stay motivated, track your advancement, and make any necessary modifications to stay on the right track.

Consult With Professionals

If it's hard for you to evaluate your current fitness level or if you feel overwhelmed by the process, seek guidance from an expert like a certified personal trainer. A professional can provide valuable insights into the feasibility of your goals and help you establish milestones along the way. Regular check-ins with a trainer can confirm that you're on the right track and offer necessary adjustments over time.

Professionals may take into account various aspects of a client's lifestyle, including their fitness history, nutrition, and work and social dynamics. These inquiries are not meant to judge but to gain a comprehensive understanding of the individual. By grasping the client's unique circumstances, a tailored program can be created to suit their specific needs and goals.

By consulting with a certified personal trainer or fitness professional, you can benefit from their expertise, receive personalized guidance, and ensure that your fitness journey is aligned with your capabilities and aspirations.

Consider Your Previous Habits

Engaging in self-reflection and asking yourself tough questions can provide valuable insights and help you determine the most suitable fitness goals for your individual circumstances.

DiSalvo suggests considering your past achievements in crushing fitness goals and whether you are ready to take it to the next level. If you have a track record of success, you might be ready to tackle more complex goals, such as running a long-distance race at a specific pace (McCoy, 2019).

However, if you are new to fitness, there is no need to worry. DiSalvo assures that focusing on simple behavior modifications is a perfectly valid approach. For instance, setting a goal of going to the gym a certain number of days per week can be an effective starting point.

Clancy emphasizes the importance of being realistic about your current fitness level and routine (McCoy, 2019). If you are not currently engaging in any form of exercise, setting a goal of going to the gym five days a week, while possible, may not be the most practical or realistic objective to begin with. It's crucial to consider your starting point and set goals that align with your current abilities.

Additionally, it is helpful to reflect on past obstacles that may have hindered your goal attainment. For example, if you struggle with morning workouts, it may be more effective to do an evening workout instead of aiming for early morning sessions. Being honest with yourself and acknowledging potential barriers upfront enables you to identify and eliminate them proactively, setting yourself up for success from the start.

By taking the time to assess your fitness history, current capabilities, and potential obstacles, you can make informed decisions about your goals, setting yourself on a path that is both practical and achievable.

Know Your Support Structure

While considering your fitness goals, it's essential to think about the individuals in your life who can provide encouragement, motivation, and accountability. Enlisting their support can make a significant difference in your journey. You can never go wrong with surrounding yourself with people who are supportive of your goals, especially those with whom you spend the most time.

By sharing your aspirations with those who will uplift and inspire you, you create a network of support that can help propel you forward. These individuals can offer words of encouragement during challenging times, provide motivation when you feel discouraged, and hold you accountable for your commitments. Their presence can make the journey more enjoyable, and their support can bolster your chances of success.

When selecting individuals to be part of your support system, choose those who genuinely believe in your abilities and are committed to helping you achieve your goals. Whether it's family members, friends, workout buddies, or even a fitness community, their positive influence and encouragement can play a vital role in keeping you motivated and on track.

Remember, you don't have to embark on your fitness journey alone. By involving and relying on the support of those around you, you can create a strong network of allies who will be there to cheer you on every step of the way.

TIPS TO KEEP IN MIND

Knowing how to set your fitness goals strategically is great, but one can never get enough tips when it comes to holistically approaching their health. Here are some valuable tips to help you on your journey to feeling healthier, happier, and more rested:

Consult With Your Physician

Although many seniors are capable of engaging in physical activity, certain conditions can impose limitations on the amount and types of exercise they can undertake. For instance, individuals with congestive heart failure or lung disease may experience difficulties with breathing, and exercise could potentially exacerbate their symptoms. Moreover, those with osteoporosis or a history of bone fractures may face an increased risk of injury during exercise.

As always, it's crucial to consult with a doctor before implementing significant changes to one's health and lifestyle. Regular checkups are customary for many senior citizens, so don't hesitate to inquire about the suitability of exercise for your specific circumstances during your next visit.

Wear Suitable Gear

Wearing ill-fitting clothing such as baggy pants, shoes that don't fit properly, or exercise gear that is too tight can potentially create safety hazards. For instance, if the clothing is excessively tight, it could strain the muscles when you move. Inadequately fitting shoes can increase the chances of falls, leading to potential bone fractures or head injuries. It's essential to wear suitable attire, even for chair exercises at home.

Warm Up and Cool Down

Incorporating warm-up and stretching exercises before a workout can help minimize the likelihood of muscle soreness. By engaging in a warm-up routine, you can elevate your body temperature and enhance blood flow to the muscles. Additionally, it's beneficial for you to allocate time for a cooling-down period following your exercise session.

Start Low and Slow

While it's important for your exercise routine to be challenging, it's equally crucial to avoid overwhelming yourself. Pushing too hard can result in muscle strains or bone fractures. It's essential for you to be aware of your body's limits and strive to stay within those boundaries. If you ever feel overexerted, it may be advisable to reduce the intensity of the exercises until you're ready to gradually increase it again.

Stick to a Schedule

To develop a lasting exercise routine, dedicate yourself to a consistent schedule for a minimum of three to four weeks. By doing so, you allow it to become a habit and increase your likelihood of sticking with it. Finding activities that you genuinely enjoy can greatly facilitate this process, as it becomes easier to stay motivated and committed.

Remember to Stretch

Don't forget to warm up to reduce sore muscles and enhance blood flow to the muscles.

Stay Hydrated

Dehydration can pose safety risks for seniors, especially during exercise. Insufficient intake of water and other healthy fluids can lead to muscle cramps, headaches, and weakness. It's important for you to drink an ample amount of water while exercising to prevent dizziness and low blood pressure.

Get a Partner

One of the essential exercise safety tips for seniors is to engage in physical activity with a partner. Exercising with another person offers several advantages. Firstly, you'll have someone to observe your form and provide encouragement throughout your workout. Secondly, having a companion serves as a valuable precautionary measure in case of accidents or falls. Unfortunately, falls are a leading cause of emergency room visits among the elderly, and having someone nearby can provide assistance and support when needed.

Don't Overdo It

Engaging in exercise when you're unwell or experiencing excessive fatigue is never a good idea. You may think that you're helping the situation, but physical activity can, in fact, worsen your illness when you are sick. You also run the risk of subjecting yourself to injury if you are excessively tired.

Have a Game Plan

You have already learned about SMART goals (Specific, Measurable, Achievable, Relevant, and Time-bound), but I will reiterate this: You need to assess your current level of fitness before embarking on a fitness journey. Based on your assessment, create a well-rounded plan that's not only safe but efficient and effective in helping you achieve your fitness goals. Stay open to changing your plan to suit your needs at any point. While success may entail 20 squats today, on a different day, you can do 50 or bring them down to just 5 (depending on your health and overall well-being).

TOOLS NEEDED

You will need a chair (preferably an armless chair), a yoga strap, and a pair of light weights.

STAYING MOTIVATED

Sticking to an exercise routine is a commitment, and just like with any other commitment, you won't always feel motivated to meet your daily or weekly goals. Unfortunately, our bodies don't stop needing exercise because we don't feel like it. On the contrary, you may need endorphins on the day you feel low more than any other day.

However, you should never feel bad for not always feeling up to the task; it's just part of human nature, and we all go through those days. You can, however, learn the strategies necessary to stay motivated so that you can continue to enhance your health and overall well-being. Let's dive right into some of those strategies.

Develop Manageable Goals

Don't be too presumptuous; I may have made that mistake myself. The problem is that setting extreme goals isn't always sustainable, and once you start slacking, you will start doubting yourself and your capabilities.

Another huge part of setting manageable goals is to avoid comparing yourself to others. While exercising with a group of like-minded people will go a long way in fueling your desire to show up for your goals each day, you may risk burnout if you move at other people's pace. Therefore, be conscious of your own capabilities and limitations, set goals that resonate with your health, and stay true to yourself.

Take Full Advantage of Technology

Many of us can relate to having a closet filled with unused ab rollers and fitness DVDs. Sadly, while new purchases are great, they won't always sustain motivation for a fitness routine.

However, there is an exception to this rule: Fitness watches, also known as wearable technology, can genuinely keep us motivated. I find that wearing a fitness watch helps me to stay accountable and motivated. Beyond simply telling time, fitness watches can track various metrics such as steps, daily activity, calories burned, heart rate, and even sleep patterns. Moreover, many fitness trackers offer built-in workouts, tips, and apps to help you set realistic goals. Research has shown that even a basic pedometer can increase activity levels by 30% (Heather, n.d).

You can also consider utilizing a fitness app for extra motivation. The good thing is that there is a wide range of apps available specifically designed for this purpose. While some apps offer motivational quotes and affirmations, others enable you to track your progress, set reminders, or even engage in friendly competitions to keep things engaging. When selecting an app, ensure that it aligns with your lifestyle and fitness level. For beginners, I recommend a user-friendly app that isn't overly complex.

Seek Fun Ways to Help You Stay Accountable

We've all been tempted to skip exercising and indulge in all our feel-good food; it's just so much easier to sit, eat, and enjoy. However, we all need to stay accountable. How else can we remain active and reach our fitness goals?

An effective strategy for staying motivated is finding a workout buddy with similar goals and schedules. You can also consider hiring a personal trainer, but I didn't have to spend money on a trainer while doing chair exercises in my own home. In my own journey, having an accountability partner has been more than helpful.

Acknowledge and Appreciate Your Accomplishments

It takes time to get results, and before that happens, it's so easy to get disheartened. However, I urge you to be patient with yourself; there is no such thing as immediate results (at least not the ones that are noticeable). When you start feeling disheartened, remind yourself that all good things take time, and instead of criticizing yourself for not reaching your desired destination, pause and appreciate the small triumphs you achieve along the journey.

I believe that every milestone is worth celebrating, regardless of size or apparent significance. One should always make it a point to take a few moments each day to acknowledge their accomplishments, even if it's as simple as waking up on time or avoiding distractions during workout sessions. When you acknowledge and celebrate small daily wins, you can greatly boost your motivation and be able to maintain it in the long run.

Make a Playlist That Makes You Want to Move

When it comes to working out, nothing can get you moving quite like some fantastic music. Scientific studies have revealed that music not only enhances endurance and exercise performance but also combats exercise fatigue (Heather, n.d.).

You can either create your own workout playlists or explore the wide selection of ready-to-go playlists available on popular apps like Spotify, Pandora, and YouTube. Additionally, you can use the Future Fitness App, as it offers a range of carefully curated playlists within the app itself, designed to keep you energized throughout your workouts.

Reward Yourself

Lastly, it's crucial to acknowledge and reward yourself for the hard work and dedication you've invested. When you reach a milestone or make significant progress in your fitness journey, take a moment to celebrate your achievements. This can be as simple as treating yourself to new workout gear, indulging in a spa day, or even taking a well-deserved break from your workout routine.

Some people don't see the significance of rewarding themselves, but it's a simple act that will go a long way. Not only will rewarding yourself allow you to recognize and value all the progress you have made in pursuit of your fitness goals, but it also acts as a source of motivation during challenging times. So, don't think twice. Reward yourself. You deserve it!

AGE IS JUST A NUMBER

Flo Filion Meiler, an 84-year-old exceptional athlete hailing from Shelburne, Vermont, accomplished remarkable success by winning multiple medals at the indoor World Masters Athletics Championships in Poland.

She secured gold medals in high jump, pentathlon, 60-meter hurdles, and pole vault, along with silver medals in long jump and triple jump. Meiler and her fellow teammates also set a new world record in the 4x200 relay for women in their 80s.

What's even more remarkable is looking at Meiler's journey in the pole vault event. At the age of 65, after watching a pole vaulting competition at the Senior Olympics, she felt inspired to take it up herself. Despite the challenge, Meiler embraced it wholeheartedly, relying on her strong upper body, core, and arms, honed through 30 years as a competitive slalom water skier.

Although she was the only pole vaulter in her age division at the world championships, Meiler noted that there were a few men competing in the 80–84 age group. She also mentioned the presence of a 103-year-old woman from India, demonstrating that age was no barrier to participation and achieving personal goals.

Flo Filion Meiler maintained a demanding training schedule to achieve her remarkable success. She dedicated five to six days a week to workouts, leaving no time for skiing, which she used to enjoy.

Her training regimen consisted of track events on Mondays, Wednesdays, and Fridays, while Tuesdays and Thursdays were dedicated to machine weights. She also engaged in doubles tennis, although it was more for socializing than intense training. While she mostly trained alone, Meiler received assistance from a coach at the University of Vermont, particularly for shot put and high jump.

Recognizing the impact of aging on her body, Meiler increased the time she spent on stretching and warming up after experiencing hamstring problems in 2018. This adjustment proved instrumental in preventing injuries. Despite the thinning competition, retirement was not on Meiler's horizon. As long as she maintained good health, she was determined to continue her athletic pursuits indefinitely.

In 2019, her focus was the Senior Olympics in Albuquerque, New Mexico. Additionally, she celebrated her birthday in June of 2019, which marked her transition to the next age bracket. Meiler was excited to be 85, as it provided an opportunity to challenge existing records and push her own limits (Wamsley, 2019).

3

CHAIR YOGA

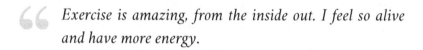 *Exercise is amazing, from the inside out. I feel so alive and have more energy.*

— VANESSA HUDGENS

Before engaging in any exercise regimen, it's crucial that you prioritize warming up and stretching to prepare your body for physical activity. Chair yoga serves as an excellent starting point as it helps you loosen up and enhance flexibility, making you ready for other exercises. By incorporating chair yoga into your routine, you can gently ease into your exercise regimen while reaping the benefits of improved mobility, relaxation, and overall well-being.

POSES FOR THE NECK

In our modern lives, stress and tension often accumulate in our heads and necks, especially for those who spend prolonged periods sitting at a computer. However, for us seniors, whether or not we spend lots of time sitting on our computers is of little relevance when it comes to neck stiffness and soreness. We can just expect it, but we can also do something about it.

Built-up tension can result in neck pain, headaches, and restricted mobility in the shoulders and head. To address this all-too-common discomfort, you can use various yoga poses specifically designed to alleviate neck pain and offer quick, soothing relief. By following these exercises, you can experience the benefits of these poses, finding relief from tension and promoting increased comfort and mobility in the neck area. Let's dive in:

Cow Face Pose

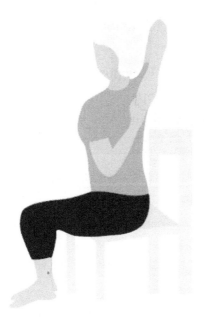

Cow Face pose is beneficial for stretching and opening the chest and shoulders.

To practice this pose:

- Begin in a comfortable seated position.
- Raise your left elbow and bend your arm, bringing your left hand towards your back.
- Use your right hand to gently pull your left elbow over to the right side, or bring your right hand up to reach and hold your left hand.
- Hold this pose for about 30 seconds, feeling a gentle stretch in your chest and shoulders.

- Repeat the same steps on the other side, raising your right elbow and bending your arm, and using your left hand to guide the stretch to the left.

By incorporating the Cow Face pose into your routine, you can effectively stretch and open your chest and shoulders, promoting improved flexibility and relieving tension in these areas.

Head Circle

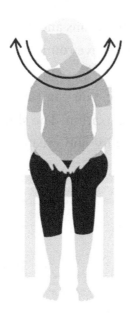

To perform this gentle neck exercise:

- Find a comfortable seated position.
- Take a moment to deepen your breath, focusing on slow and steady inhales and exhales.
- Drop your right ear towards your right shoulder, feeling a stretch on the left side of your neck.
- Gently roll your head to the center and then tilt your left ear towards your left shoulder, stretching the right side of your neck.
- Throughout the exercise, keep your eyes closed and your gaze inward, directed towards your third eye center.

- Move your head in gentle and slow circles, completing about five rounds in one direction.
- Afterward, switch directions and continue the movement for another five rounds.

By practicing this exercise, you can find relief from tension in the neck and promote relaxation. The slow and mindful circles help improve neck mobility and create a sense of inner focus and calmness.

Neck Releasing Pose

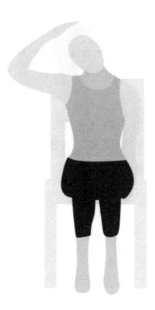

Please note that this stretch is not recommended if you have bulging disks or other neck problems.

- Grab onto the chair edge with your left hand.
- Ensure that you maintain a gentle grip without exerting excessive pressure.
- If you are sitting on a bench or couch, extend your left fingers out to the left, placing them on the seat.
- Reach your right arm overhead and touch your left ear with your fingertips.
- Gently tilt you right ear towards your right shoulder without applying pressure.
- If you are holding onto the chair seat, maintain your grip and lean your body slightly to the right, allowing for a deeper stretch on the left side of your neck.

- If you are not holding onto the chair seat, continue walking your left fingers to the left until you feel a stretch along the left side of your neck.
- Stay in this position for approximately 30 seconds, and then switch to the opposite side.

It's important to remember that if you have any neck issues or concerns, it's advisable to consult with a healthcare professional before attempting this stretch.

Shoulder Opener

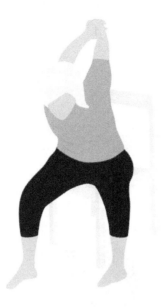

The following stretch can be done either seated or standing. Here are the steps:

- Begin by positioning your feet wider than your hips.
- Grasp a belt, scarf, or towel behind you, keeping your hands shoulder-width apart. Don't despair if you don't have props; simply link your fingers together at the bottom of your lower back.
- Fold forward, allowing your arms to extend behind you, reaching towards the sky to open up your shoulders.
- Hold this position for about 20–30 seconds, feeling the stretch in your shoulders and hamstrings.
- Return back to the center position.

Incorporating these chair exercises into your routine can be highly beneficial for maintaining flexibility and overall well-being.

Triceps Shoulder Stretch

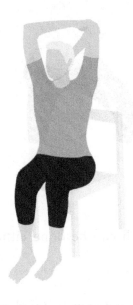

While seated at the edge of your chair, follow these steps for the stretch:

- Raise your right arm up towards the sky.
- Bend your right elbow and bring your right hand towards your upper back.
- Rest your left hand on your right elbow.
- Gently press your right elbow into your left hand.
- Simultaneously, gently press your left hand into your right elbow.

- Focus on lengthening the space between your right shoulder and right elbow as much as possible.
- Hold this position for approximately 30 seconds.
- Then, switch to the opposite side and repeat the stretch.
- Finally, return to the center position.

By performing this stretch, you can effectively target the muscles in your shoulders and promote improved flexibility and range of motion. Remember to listen to your body and avoid any discomfort or pain during the stretch.

Seated Cat

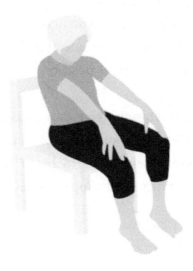

This exercise will alleviate tension in your neck and back. To practice, follow the steps below:

- Place your palms on your knees or lap.
- Hold onto the kneecaps and straighten your arms.
- Round your back and simultaneously lean back, directing your gaze towards your navel.
- Spread out your scapulae (shoulder blades) to the sides while allowing your shoulders and neck to relax.
- Take a long, deep breath in, and exhale slowly and steadily for three breaths.
- To release the stretch, inhale and return your spine to an upright position, and exhale.

Avoid this stretch if you experience any pain in the neck.

Upper Back Eagle Arm Stretch

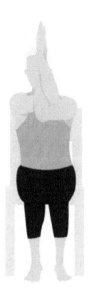

Sit at the front of your chair and follow these steps for the stretch (ensure your feet are hip-width apart):

- Extend your arms straight in front of you, aligning them with your shoulders.
- Place your right elbow on top of the left elbow and interlace your forearms. Alternatively, if interlacing is uncomfortable, cross your arms and hold onto the opposite shoulders with your hands.
- Press your forearms or elbows forward while simultaneously widening your upper back. Separate your shoulder blades, directing your heart area toward the wall behind you.
- You can choose to remain in this position or gently curl your elbows inward toward your stomach.

- Take slow, deep breaths, focusing on releasing any tension in your upper back and neck.
- Hold this stretch for 30 to 60 seconds, then switch your arms, placing the left elbow on top of the right.
- Return to the center position.

This stretch aims to relieve tightness in the upper back and shoulders. Remember to listen to your body and modify the stretch if needed to ensure your comfort and safety.

POSES FOR THE CORE AND ARMS

Chair yoga offers a convenient way to alleviate tension, reduce stress, and cultivate a sense of well-being and equilibrium. Incorporating upper body stretches into your daily routine can help alleviate tension, boost energy levels, or promote relaxation during hectic moments. These gentle exercises can easily be integrated into your day for optimal benefits:

Hand, Wrist, and Elbow Rescue

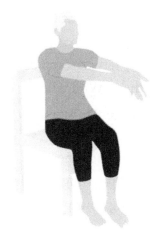

These stretches can be done while seated, providing relief and promoting flexibility in your hands, wrists, and elbows. Remember to move slowly and listen to your body, only stretching to a comfortable level (Blick, 2017).

Hands:

- Start by facing your palms towards each other, with your fingertips touching.
- Slowly stretch your fingers apart, creating space between them.
- Press your palms toward each other, feeling a gentle stretch in the spaces between your fingers and the backs of your hands.

Wrist/Elbow:

- Extend your right arm forward, palm facing upward, and ensure that your elbow is straight.
- Reach out with your left arm and bring your palms together, joining them. While doing so, softly push your right fingers towards the floor, experiencing a gentle stretch in your wrist and elbow.
- Repeat this stretch on the other side, extending your left arm forward and pressing your left fingers toward the floor while joining your palms together.

Torso, Back, and Shoulder Flow

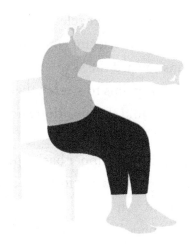

Incorporating these stretches into your routine can enhance your upper body mobility, relieve tension, and promote a sense of well-being. Remember to listen to your body and modify the movements as needed for your comfort (Blick, 2017).

- Link your fingers together before rotating your palms so they face outward.
- Take a deep breath and extend your arms, pushing your palms forward while stretching your torso forward.
- Lift your torso upright and raise your hands overhead.
- Exhale as your arms gracefully float down to your sides.
- Repeat the above sequence three to five times to promote flexibility and relaxation.

For the final repetition:

- Engage in a torso and shoulder release by holding your arms above your head, interlacing your fingers, and turning your palms toward the sky.
- Push up through your palms to stretch the front of your shoulders and chest. Hold this position and feel the gentle release.
- Begin the transition into an upper back opening position by extending your arms forward and pushing your palms in front of you.
- Gently curve your upper back, tuck your chin in, and proceed to shift your hands from side to side.
- Experience a stretch behind and between your shoulder blades, and hold this position to encourage openness in your upper back.

Energizing Backbend, Chest Opener

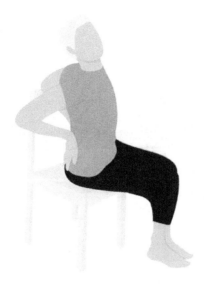

- Grab your hips with your hands.
- Take a deep inhale as you lift your chest up, extending your spine.
- Gently look up, allowing your neck to lengthen.
- Pull your elbows back, opening your shoulders and expanding your chest.
- Hold this posture, feeling the stretch and openness in your upper body.

By practicing this stretch, you can improve your posture, release tension, and promote a sense of openness and confidence. Remember to breathe deeply throughout the movement and adjust the intensity according to your comfort level.

Chair Eagle—Garudasana

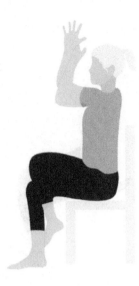

- Start by crossing your right thigh over your left thigh, creating a figure-four shape for the Eagle Pose.
- If possible, try to wrap your right foot around the left calf while keeping your balance and stability.
- Bring your left arm across the right one at the elbow, aligning your palms to meet and touch.
- Bend the elbows, lifting them while simultaneously dropping your shoulders away from the ears.
- Hold this position for three to five breaths, feeling the stretch and engagement in your upper body.
- Repeat the sequence on the other side, crossing the left thigh over the right thigh and wrapping the left foot around the right calf.
- Cross your right arm over the left one at the elbow, bringing the palms together.

- Lift the elbows, relax the shoulders, and hold for
  another three to five breaths.

Eagle Pose is a great way to improve balance, flexibility, and focus. Remember to listen to your body and modify the pose as needed to ensure a comfortable and safe experience.

Seated Mountain

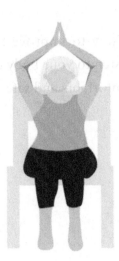

To practice this pose, follow these steps:

- Begin by sitting on the front half of your chair, ensuring your back is straight, and your core is engaged.
- Bend your knees at 90-degree angles, making sure your knees are positioned above your ankles, and maintain a small gap between your knees.
- Raise your hands up over your head, with your palms together and your elbows slightly bent.
- Inhale slowly, and as you exhale, roll your shoulders downward, allowing any tension to release.
- Activate your abdominal muscles, drawing them gently inward, and keep your arms relaxed at your sides.
- Hold this pose for several deep breaths, focusing on maintaining proper alignment and allowing yourself to feel grounded and centered.

Enjoy the benefits of this seated posture for relaxation and strengthening your core muscles.

Side Bend/Half-Moon

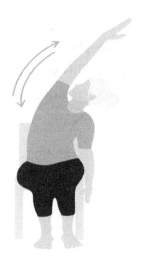

To perform this sequence, follow these steps:

- Inhale deeply and reach your right arm up while simultaneously lowering your left arm down.
- Lift and lengthen your spine, maintaining a tall posture.
- Exhale as you gently bend your torso towards the left, ensuring that your shoulders remain squared.
- Hold this position, feeling a stretch along the right side of your body.
- Continue the sequence on the right side by taking a deep breath in, extending your left arm upward, and lowering your right arm downward.

- Once again, lift and elongate your spine, then exhale as you gently lean your torso to the right while keeping your shoulders aligned.
- Hold this position until you feel a stretch along your left side.

Remember to breathe deeply throughout the sequence and listen to your body's limits. This stretch helps to release tension and promote flexibility in your side body.

Seated Forward Bend

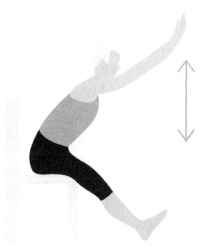

- Sit facing forward, maintaining a comfortable distance of about two arm's lengths from your desk.
- Extend your legs, hip distance apart, and ensure that your heels are firmly on the ground.
- Inhale deeply as you raise your arms from your sides up towards the sky. Roll your shoulders away from your ears, moving them down and back.
- Gaze upwards towards your palms.
- Keeping your spine straight and your arms extended, slowly exhale as you bend forward from your waist, bringing your upper body over your legs.
- Allow your hands to rest on the floor and let your head hang loosely and heavily between your knees.

Benefits:

- It relieves tension in the neck caused by prolonged screen time.
- It reduces stress on the neck muscles and upper spine caused by the weight of the head.
- It provides a deep stretch for the lower back, promoting relaxation and relieving tension in the lumbar spine.

By incorporating this pose into your routine, you can address the strains and tensions that result from extended periods of sitting and screen use. Remember to breathe deeply and listen to your body's limits as you perform this stretch.

Overhead Stretch (Chair Raised Hands Pose—Urdhva Hastasana)

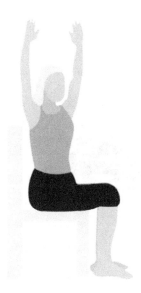

- Sit upright in your chair.
- Relax your shoulders and ensure that your rib cage is aligned naturally over your hips.
- On an inhalation, raise your arms upward toward the ceiling.
- Keep your sit bones anchored to the chair seat and reach up from that stable base.
- On an exhalation, lower your arms down and return to the starting position.
- Repeat the exercise for 3-5 times.

By practicing this stretch, you can promote good posture and engage your upper body muscles. Remember to breathe deeply and maintain a relaxed state throughout the exercise.

Cat and Cow Stretch

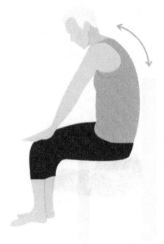

To perform this seated spinal stretch, follow these steps:

- Sit comfortably in your chair with your feet touching the ground.
- Maintain a straight spine, chin slightly up, with shoulders back.
- Place your hands and palms down on your thighs.
- Proceed to breathe in slowly as you arch your spine while simultaneously moving your hands down to your knees.
- Pay attention to your body's sensations as you begin to feel relaxed and free of tension.
- Breathe out slowly as you create a circle-like posture with your spine by tucking your chin toward your chest and bringing your head and shoulders forward.

- Slowly return your hands to the starting position, lift your head, and straighten your spine.
- You can practice this exercise at least five times.

By practicing this sequence, you can promote flexibility and mobility in your spine while also bringing awareness to your breath.

Chair Spinal Twist

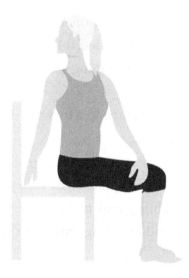

To perform a seated spinal twist on a chair, follow these steps:

- Sit sideways on the chair, with your body facing towards the right. Keep your feet flat on the floor and your spine long.
- Twist your torso toward the right, reaching for the back of the chair with your hands. Allow your gaze to follow the twist.

- As you inhale, lengthen your spine by sitting tall and engaging your core muscles.
- On each exhale, deepen the twist by gently rotating your torso further to the right. Feel the stretch along your spine.
- Continue this lengthening and twisting motion for five breaths, maintaining a steady and relaxed breathing pattern.
- After completing the twist on the right side, shift your legs around to the left side of the chair.
- Repeat the same twisting motion, this time twisting your torso toward the left side. Hold the twist for five breaths, focusing on maintaining good posture and a smooth breath.
- Release the twist and return to a forward-facing position on the chair.

By incorporating this seated spinal twist into your routine, you can help improve flexibility and mobility in your spine while promoting relaxation and releasing tension in your upper body.

Triangle Pose

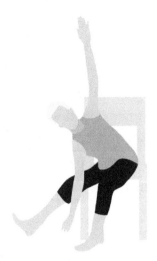

Triangle Pose, also known as Trikonasana, is an effective position for relieving pain and tension in the neck, shoulders, and upper back. Follow these steps to practice Triangle Pose:

- Begin by sitting with your feet wider than hip-width apart. You can jump, step, or walk your feet apart to achieve the desired width.
- Stretch your right leg out while keeping right heel firmly on the ground and your toes pointing upward. Keep your left toes facing outwards at a comfortable angle.
- Extend your arms out to the sides, parallel to the floor, with your palms facing down.
- Keeping your legs engaged, reach forward with your right arm, hinging at your right thigh. Your left arm should be lifted up toward the ceiling.

- Find a comfortable position for your gaze, either looking in any direction or performing gentle neck rotations by looking up and down.
- Maintain the pose for about 30 seconds, focusing on your breath and allowing the stretch to release tension in your neck, shoulders, and upper back.
- To transition to the other side, slowly bring your left arm down and lift your right arm as you rotate your feet. Repeat the steps on the opposite side, maintaining balance and alignment.

By incorporating Triangle Pose into your practice, you can experience relief from pain and tension in your upper body while improving strength, flexibility, and overall posture.

Chair Warrior I—Virabhadrasana I

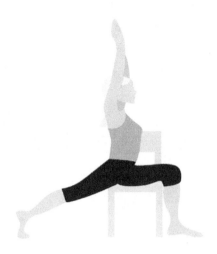

Chair Warrior Pose, also known as Chair Virabhadrasana, is a modified version of the traditional Warrior Pose that can be practiced while seated. This pose offers numerous benefits, including improved strength, stability, and focus. Here's how you can practice Chair Warrior Pose (Pizer, 2022):

- Make sure your hips are squared to face forward.
- While your left leg is firmly placed on the ground, put your right leg far behind you.
- Straighten the right leg and place the toes firmly on the ground.
- While keeping your upper body facing the left leg, raise your arms towards the ceiling as you inhale, entering the Warrior I pose.
- Hold the Warrior I pose for three breaths, focusing on your alignment and grounding through your legs.

This exercise strengthens the arms, shoulders, and core muscles while stretching and opening the sides of the body. It can also improve balance and concentration. Whether you're at work, in a meeting, or at home, practicing Chair Warrior Pose can provide a rejuvenating break and promote a sense of grounding and empowerment.

Chair Warrior II

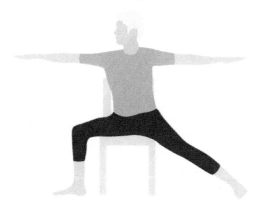

Chair Warrior II is a pose that can help open and strengthen your chest and shoulders, providing support for your neck. Here's how to practice it (Pizer, 2022):

- Exhale and open up the arms, extending the left arm forward and the right arm back.
- Move your right hip back and rotate your torso to the right, aligning it with the front of the chair.
- Maintain a steady gaze over left fingertips, focusing on a point in the distance.
- Hold the Warrior II pose for three breaths, feeling the strength and stability in your legs and the expansion in your chest and shoulder. (*please note the image above shows the exercise performed for the right side*).

Chair Warrior II helps to create space and strength in the chest and shoulders, offering support and relief for the neck. It also promotes stability, balance, and a sense of groundedness.

Regular practice of Chair Warrior II can enhance your posture and bring a greater sense of openness and strength to your upper body.

Reverse Warrior

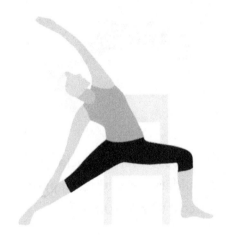

Reverse Warrior is a yoga pose that provides a deep stretch while building strength in the legs and core. Here's how to practice it:

- Exhale while lowering your right arm down the left leg. Inhale while reaching your left arm up toward the ceiling to create the Reverse Warrior pose. Hold this position for three breaths, feeling the stretch along the right side of your body.
- After finishing Reverse Warrior on the left side, bring both legs to the front of the chair.

- Sit sideways on the chair, facing right, and repeat the series of three warrior poses (Warrior I, Warrior II, Reverse Warrior) on the right side.
- Remember to maintain proper alignment and focus on your breath throughout the poses.

Reverse Warrior is a powerful pose that promotes flexibility, strength, and balance. It helps to increase mobility in the spine, stretch the intercostal muscles, and open up the chest and shoulders. Regular practice of Reverse Warrior can enhance your overall body awareness and bring a sense of vitality and energy to your practice.

POSES FOR FEET AND TOES

Heel Raise

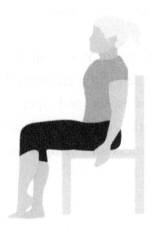

- Sit on the chair with your feet positioned at right angles to your knees, creating a 90-degree angle resembling two pillars. Ensure that your calves are perpendicular to the floor.
- Begin by lifting your right heel off the ground while keeping the left heel grounded. Take notice of all the sensations and bones in your feet as you hold this position for a few seconds.
- Alternate between lifting your right and left heels, continuing to observe the sensations and movements in your feet. Allow your breath to flow naturally throughout the exercise. Repeat this movement 10 times.

This exercise stimulates blood flow to the feet and calves, promoting healthy circulation and potentially preventing varicose veins. Additionally, it activates the reflex zones in the feet, which can have a relaxing effect on the entire spine, potentially assisting with various back problems.

Rocking the Feet

- Sit comfortably on the chair with both feet flat on the floor.
- Begin by lifting your toes off the ground while keeping your heels grounded. Feel the stretch and engagement in the muscles of your feet.
- Next, lower your toes and lift your heels off the ground, shifting the weight onto the balls of your feet. Notice the change in sensation and the activation of different muscles.
- Continue alternating between raising your toes and heels, creating a gentle rocking motion. Repeat this movement 5 to 10 times.

Benefits: This exercise helps to loosen the musculature of the feet, providing relief and relaxation to the foot and hip joints. It can also improve circulation and enhance overall foot mobility.

Rolling the Feet

- Sit with your feet shoulder-width apart, ensuring a stable stance.
- Start by rolling your feet inwards, shifting the weight to the inner edges of your feet. Feel the stretch and activation along the inner arches and ankles.
- Gradually roll your feet outwards, transferring the weight to the outer edges of your feet. Notice the engagement in the outer arches and ankles.
- Continue rolling your feet inwards and outwards, smoothly transitioning between the inner and outer edges. Pay attention to the sensations in your feet, toes, and ankles.
- Repeat this rolling motion for a few rounds, allowing the movement to flow naturally.

This exercise enhances circulation to the feet and calves, promoting healthy blood flow. It also helps to improve the flexibility and mobility of the feet, providing a sense of relief and relaxation.

Flex and Stretch

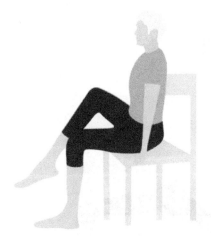

- Begin by raising your right foot off the ground.
- Take a deep inhale and flex your entire foot, pulling your toes towards you.
- Exhale and point your toes away from you, extending your foot forward.
- Repeat this flex-and-point movement three times, allowing your breath to guide the rhythm.
- After completing the repetitions, proceed to circle your right ankle clockwise several times.
- Then, circle your right ankle counterclockwise for the same number of rotations.
- Lower your right foot back to the ground and repeat the entire sequence with your left foot.

This exercise helps to loosen the ankles, enhancing their flexibility and range of motion. Additionally, the synchronized movements and deep breathing promote increased circulation to the feet, ankles, and calves, supporting overall foot health.

Chair Extended Side Angle

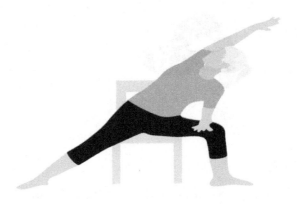

- Begin by bending forward from the hips, allowing your upper body to fold down.
- Place your left hand on the left side of your thigh for support.
- Take a deep inhalation, opening your chest and twisting your torso to the right.
- As you twist, raise your right arm up towards the ceiling and direct your gaze upward.
- Hold this position for several breaths, maintaining a steady and relaxed breath.
- If reaching the floor with your hand feels challenging, you can elevate your foot by using blocks or a prop for support, allowing for an easier twist at a higher level.
- After holding the twist on the right side, release the twist and repeat the same sequence on the left side.

- Alternate between twisting to the right and left, performing the same position, and synchronized breathing.

Glute Stretch

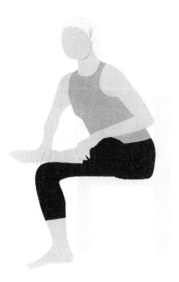

- Sit up straight in your chair.
- Cross your right ankle over your left thigh, aiming for alignment between your knee and ankle.
- Repeat the same process with your left leg, crossing your left ankle over your right thigh.
- Maintain a straight and tall posture, finding a comfortable position for your legs.
- Hold this pose, known as Chair Pigeon, for up to five breaths, focusing on steady and deep breathing.
- Feel the stretch in your hips and outer thighs while keeping a sense of relaxation.

- Release the pose gently and return to a neutral seated position when you're ready.

Hamstring Stretch

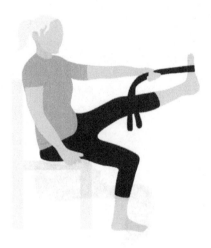

- Prepare a strap or belt to create a loop for your right foot.
- Secure the strap around your right foot and hold it in your right hand.
- Hold onto the chair edge with your other hand.
- Keep your back straight.
- Straighten and lift your right leg, keeping your back straight.
- While in the pose, you have the option to point and flex your foot a few times to engage your calf muscles and promote circulation.
- For an added challenge, slightly loosen the strap to engage your hip flexor muscles in order to maintain the lifted leg.

- Take a couple of breaths in the pose, paying attention to the sensations in your body.
- Gently lower your right foot back to the floor and take a moment to observe any changes or sensations.
- Repeat the same sequence on the other side, using the strap and lifting your left leg.
- Remember to breathe deeply and listen to your body throughout the practice.

Single Leg Forward Bend

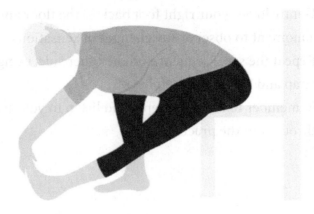

- Take the front edge of your seat.
- Place your right foot on the floor.
- Extend your left leg forward.
- Take a deep breath, lengthen your spine, and engage your core by drawing the lower belly in.
- As you exhale, gently fold forward over your outstretched leg, aiming to keep your spine long and your posture aligned.
- Extend your left hand forward and reach out to grab your toe (pay attention to your comfort level).
- Hold this position for a few breaths, allowing the stretch to deepen.
- Inhale to slowly come back to an upright seated position and bring your left foot flat on the floor.
- Take a pause for a few breaths, noticing the effects of the stretch in your body and the sensations you experience.

- When you're ready, repeat the sequence on the other side by switching the position of your legs.
- Maintain focus on your breath and body awareness throughout the practice.
- Respect your body's limits and adjust the intensity of the stretch according to your comfort level.

Seated Hero's Pose—Virasana

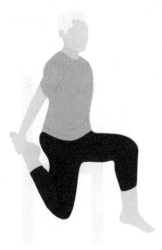

- Position yourself at the side of your chair, ensuring that your right leg is off the chair.
- Support yourself by using your left hand to hold onto the edge of the chair.
- Lean gently towards the left side as you bend your right knee.
- Reach with your right hand to hold onto your right foot, using a strap if necessary to assist your grip.
- Slowly bring your right heel towards your buttock, focusing on feeling the stretch in the front of your thigh.
- Pay attention to your body, and if you experience any discomfort or strain in your knee, release your foot slightly.
- Hold this position for a few breaths, allowing the stretch to deepen.

- Maintain a relaxed and steady breathing pattern throughout the pose.
- When you're ready, gently release the hold on your foot and return your right leg to a neutral position.
- Take a moment to notice the effects of the stretch on your body.
- Repeat the sequence on the other side, shifting to the opposite side of the chair and performing the pose with your left leg.

Chair Yoga Lunge Pose

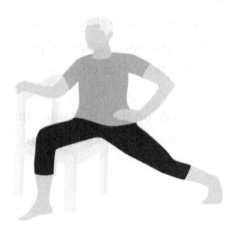

- Sit at the edge of your chair.
- Place your feet on the floor.
- Place your hands on your thighs or the sides of the chair for support and stability.
- Inhale deeply, and as you exhale, take a step forward with your right foot, extending it in front of you.
- Keep your right knee bent at a 90-degree angle, ensuring that it is aligned above your ankle and not extending beyond it.
- Extend your left leg behind you, with your toes on the ground and your heel facing upwards.
- Apply strong pressure to your right foot, activating the muscles in your leg.
- As you hold the lunge position, maintain an upright posture, with your spine tall and your shoulders relaxed.

- Take deep, steady breaths, allowing your body to relax into the stretch.
- You should feel a gentle stretch in the muscles of your left hip flexor and the front of your left thigh.
- Hold the pose for a few breaths, enjoying the stretch and focusing on your breath.
- To release, gently bring your right foot back to the starting position, returning to a seated position with both feet on the floor.
- Take a moment to rest and observe any sensations in your body.
- Repeat the same sequence on the other side, stepping forward with your left foot.

Chair Yoga Lunge Pose provides similar benefits to a standing lunge pose but with the added support and stability of the chair. It helps to improve leg strength, increase hip flexibility, and enhance balance. Regular practice of this pose can also help relieve tension in the hips and lower body, making it beneficial for those who spend long periods sitting or have limited mobility.

Remember to listen to your body and modify the pose as needed to suit your comfort level and any physical limitations you may have.

Half-Splits Pose with a Chair

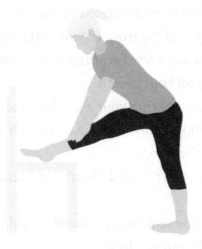

Chair Yoga Half-Splits Pose is a standing variation that focuses on balance and proprioception.

Here's how to practice Chair Yoga Half-Splits Pose:

- Start with your left leg standing firmly on the ground and your right foot resting on the chair.
- Straighten your right leg.
- Find your balance and stability in the standing leg. You can choose to stay in this position and work on improving your balance.
- While bending forward, flex your right foot by pulling your toes towards you, intensifying the stretch in the back of your leg.
- Take a few deep breaths, allowing your body to relax and sink deeper into the stretch.

- Slowly come back to an upright position, lifting your torso and bringing your hands back to your thigh or the sides of the chair.
- Take a moment to breathe and center yourself before lowering your right foot back to the floor.
- Repeat the same sequence on the other side, with your right foot standing on the ground and your left foot resting on the chair.

Chair Yoga Half-Splits Pose helps to improve balance, enhance body awareness, and increase flexibility in the back of the leg. It offers a modified version of the traditional half-splits pose, allowing individuals with limited mobility or those who prefer seated exercises to experience similar benefits.

Always listen to your body and modify the pose as necessary to accommodate your comfort level and physical abilities. If you experience any discomfort or pain, ease out of the pose and consult with a qualified yoga instructor or healthcare professional.

AGE IS JUST A NUMBER

Tao Porchon-Lynch, the world's oldest yoga teacher, passed away at the age of 101. Known for her vibrant spirit, inspiring teachings, and remarkable achievements in yoga and ballroom dancing, she left a lasting impact on her students and followers. Porchon-Lynch began her yoga journey at a young age and studied with renowned teachers throughout her life. In addition to yoga, she pursued various creative endeavors, including ballroom dancing, where she held the Guinness World Record as the oldest competitive dancer. She also had a passion for wildlife conservation and social justice, and her memoir, *Reflections: The Yogic Journey of Life*, reflects her profound wisdom. Porchon- Lynch continued to teach yoga into her 100s, showcasing her grace, strength, and stamina. Her positive outlook on aging and her belief in the cycle of life serve as an inspiration to all.

4

CARDIO EXERCISES

 Exercise should be regarded as a tribute to the heart.

— GENE TUNNERY

WARM UP

Arm Circle

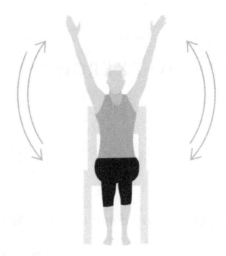

This exercise can be done in seated or lying positions, providing flexibility and versatility.

Seated Position:

- Sit upright with your arms extended straight out to the sides, forming a right angle with your body.
- Begin rotating your hands in circular motions, starting with small circles and gradually increasing their size.
- Keep your arms extended and maintain a steady rhythm as you continue the circular movements.
- Aim to perform this exercise for a duration of up to a minute, focusing on the engagement of your arms and shoulders.

Lying Position:

- Lie on your back and extend your arm up towards the ceiling.
- Start making circular motions with your hand, keeping your arm extended and maintaining a steady pace.
- After a minute, switch to the other arm and repeat the circular movements.
- Pay attention to the sensations in your arms and shoulders as you engage in this exercise.
- Remember to listen to your body and adjust the size and speed of the circles according to your comfort level.

Arm Cross

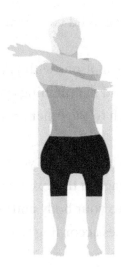

Arm Cross is a simple exercise that helps stretch and activate the muscles of your shoulders, chest, and upper back. It can be done while seated or standing.

- Sit up straight with your feet planted firmly on the ground.
- Extend your arms out to the sides at shoulder height, parallel to the floor, forming a "T" shape.
- Cross your right arm over your left one before bringing your palms together in front of your chest.
- Breathe out while uncrossing your arms and assuming the starting position.
- Repeat the movement, this time crossing your left arm over your right arm, again bringing your palms together.

- Continue alternating the cross of your arms with each breath, creating a flowing and rhythmic motion.
- Repeat this exercise for several repetitions, aiming to find a comfortable range of motion without straining.
- As you perform the Arm Cross, pay attention to the stretch and activation in your shoulders, chest, and upper back.

The Arm Cross exercise can be incorporated into your daily routine as a quick way to relieve tension and improve mobility in your upper body. It is especially beneficial for those who spend long periods sitting or working at a desk, as it helps counteract the effects of rounded shoulders and hunching forward.

Knee Open

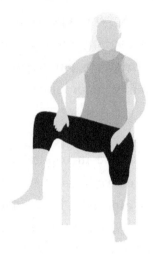

Knee Open is a seated exercise that promotes flexibility and mobility in the knees and hips.

- Begin by sitting on a chair with feet firmly on the ground. Place your hands on your thighs or knees for support and stability.
- Take a deep breath in and lengthen your spine, sitting up tall.
- On an exhale, gently push your right knee open outward, aiming to open the hip and create a stretch in the inner thigh and groin area.
- Avoid forcing the stretch or causing any pain. Instead, focus on maintaining a comfortable stretch that allows you to relax into the pose.
- Hold the position for 20–30 seconds, breathing deeply and allowing the stretch to deepen gradually.

- To release the stretch, slowly bring your right knee back and return your foot to the floor.
- Repeat the same sequence with the left knee.
- Throughout the exercise, keep your breath steady and maintain proper alignment of your spine and hips.

Knee Open is a gentle yet effective exercise that helps improve flexibility in the knees and hips. Regular practice can increase the range of motion, relieve stiffness, and promote better joint health. It is particularly beneficial for individuals who experience tightness in the inner thighs and hips, as well as those who want to maintain or improve their overall leg flexibility.

Knee Lift

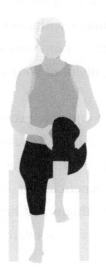

Knee Lift is a simple exercise that targets the muscles in your thighs and helps improve leg strength and stability. It can be performed while standing or seated, making it accessible for individuals with varying levels of mobility.

- Sit comfortably on a chair with your feet flat on the floor and your back straight.
- Place your hands on the sides of the chair or on your thighs for support.
- Engage your core muscles to maintain stability.
- Lift your right foot off the floor, bending your knee and bringing it towards your chest as much as you comfortably can.
- Hold the lifted position for a few seconds, focusing on maintaining balance and control.
- Gradually lower your right foot to the floor.

- Repeat the same movement with your left foot, lifting your knee towards your chest and then lowering it back down.
- Continue alternating between your right and left legs for a desired number of repetitions or times.

The Knee Lift exercise helps strengthen the quadriceps muscles in your thighs, which are essential for walking, climbing stairs, and maintaining overall leg strength. It also improves balance and stability, which can be beneficial for preventing falls and enhancing functional movements in daily activities.

Remember to start with a comfortable range of motion and gradually increase the intensity as your strength and flexibility improve. If you have any existing knee or leg conditions, it is recommended to consult with a healthcare professional before performing this exercise to ensure it is suitable for your specific needs.

EXERCISES TO GET THE HEART PUMPING

Alternating Side Reach High

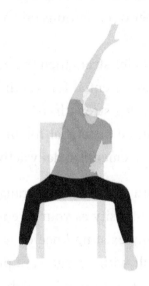

Alternating Side Reach helps improve upper body flexibility and strength. Here are the steps:

- Sit comfortably on a chair with your feet flat on the floor and your back straight.
- Place your hands on the armrests or on your thighs.
- Lift your right arm and reach it diagonally across your body towards the left side while your left arm rests on your waist.
- Extend your arm as far as you can while keeping your back straight.
- Return your right arm to the starting position.

- Repeat the movement with your left arm, reaching diagonally towards the right side.
- Continue alternating sides, reaching and returning to the starting position with each arm.
- Maintain a controlled and smooth motion, focusing on the stretch and engagement of the muscles.
- Perform the exercise for a desired number of repetitions or for a specified duration.

Remember to breathe deeply and maintain proper posture throughout the exercise.

Alternating Side Reach Low

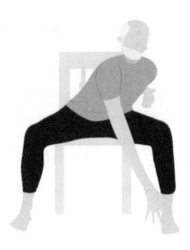

Here are the steps to follow:

- Sit comfortably on a chair with your feet flat on the floor and your back straight.
- Place your hands on the armrests or on your thighs.
- Begin by reaching your right hand down towards the left side of the chair, aiming to touch your left foot or ankle.
- Keep your back straight and avoid any twisting or leaning of your body.
- Take your right hand back to its initial position.
- Repeat the movement with your left hand, reaching down towards the right side of the chair.
- Alternate sides, reaching and returning to the starting position with each hand.
- Focus on engaging your core muscles and maintaining stability throughout the exercise.

- Perform the exercise in a controlled manner, avoiding any sudden or jerky movements.
- Continue the alternating side reaches for a desired number of repetitions or for a specified duration.

Remember to listen to your body, start with a comfortable range of motion, and gradually increase the intensity as you become more comfortable with the exercise.

Alternating V Step

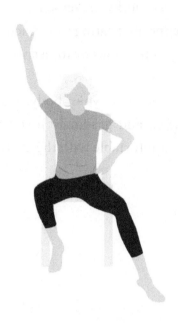

Alternating V Step helps improve cardiovascular fitness and lower body strength. It simulates the movement of a traditional V-step exercise performed on a step platform. Here are the steps:

- Sit comfortably on a chair with your feet flat on the floor and your back straight.
- Begin by lifting your right foot off the floor and stepping it out to the right side, forming a "V" shape with your legs.
- As you step out, simultaneously raise your left hand up towards the ceiling, reaching diagonally across your body.
- Return your right foot to the starting position while lowering your left hand back down.

- Now, lift your left foot off the floor and step it out to the left side, forming the other side of the "V" shape.
- As you step out to the left, raise your right hand up towards the ceiling, reaching diagonally across your body.
- Return your left foot to the starting position while lowering your right hand back down.
- Continue alternating the stepping motion, moving your feet out to the sides in a V shape while simultaneously reaching with the opposite hand.

This exercise is great for increasing heart rate. It helps improve lower body strength, coordination, and overall cardiovascular endurance.

Alternating Cross Body Knee Reach

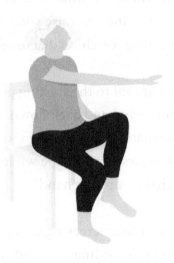

This exercise targets the core muscles and improves balance and coordination.

- While sitting in your chair, ensure that your feet are flat on the floor and your back is straight.
- Start by lifting your right knee towards your chest, bringing it up as high as possible.
- At the same time, extend your left arm diagonally across your body, reaching toward the lifted knee.
- Pause for a moment, feeling the contraction in your abdominal muscles.
- Lower your right leg back to the starting position while bringing your left arm back to the side.
- Repeat the same movement on the other side, lifting your left knee towards your chest and reaching your right arm diagonally across your body.

Seated Hinge and Cross

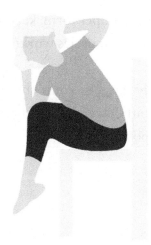

Here are the steps for a chair exercise routine that strengthens your abs, back muscles, and lower body:

- Sit upright on a chair with your knees together and your feet flat on the floor.
- Point your toes and lift your hands, bringing them behind your head.
- Engage your abdominal muscles by bracing them.
- Lean back slightly, ensuring that your shoulder blades lightly touch the back of the chair.
- Cross your right elbow towards your left knee, bringing them together in the center.
- Slowly return to the starting position.
- Switch sides and repeat the movement, crossing your left elbow towards your right knee.
- Continue alternating sides, performing a total of 20 reps (10 reps on each side).

- Maintain controlled and deliberate movements throughout the exercise.
- Focus on maintaining proper form, keeping your core engaged, and feeling the muscles working.

This routine effectively targets your abs and back muscles while also engaging your lower body. It enhances your core strength, stability, and posture.

Alternating Cross Body Toe Touch

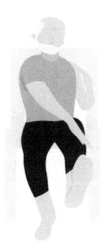

- Sit upright on a chair with your feet flat on the floor and knees together.
- Stretch your arms forward, keeping them parallel to the floor.
- Keep your abs engaged and maintain good posture throughout the exercise.
- Lift your right leg off the floor and simultaneously twist your torso to bring your left hand towards your right foot.
- Aim to touch your right foot with your left hand or reach as close as you comfortably can.
- Go back to the initial position and replicate the movement on the opposite side.
- Aim to perform 10 to 12 repetitions on each side or as many as you can comfortably do.

This exercise targets your obliques, abdominal muscles, and hip flexors while also promoting spinal mobility and stretching the hamstrings.

Seated Jacks

Seated Jacks are a great exercise that can be performed without leaving your chair. They provide a cardio- vascular workout and help you burn calories. Here's how to do seated jacks:

- Sit straight in your chair with your knees held together and your toes pointed.
- Keep your elbows straight and your arms open at the sides.
- Ensure that your palms are facing forward.
- Extend both legs out to the sides while flexing your feet.
- Let your legs land on your heels and bring both arms together overhead, resembling a regular jumping jack motion.
- Go back to your initial position.
- Try to do 20–30 reps of this exercise.

Skater Switch

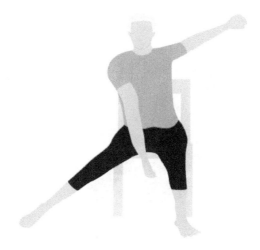

- Sit at the edge of your chair.
- Try to keep your knee bent as you extend your right leg out (as illustrated).
- Your toes should point forward throughout the exercise.
- Extend your arms and lean forward, reaching toward the inside of your left foot with your right hand.
- Switch sides quickly, reaching toward the inside of your right foot with your left arm.
- Rest and repeat the movement.
- Aim to perform 25–30 alternating repetitions.

This exercise provides a calorie-burning workout while engaging various muscle groups such as the core, inner thighs, arms, and shoulders. It is an effective way to strengthen and tone these areas without putting excessive strain on your joints.

Shadow Boxing

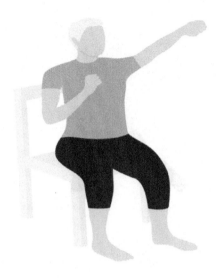

- Sit comfortably in the chair with your feet planted firmly on the floor.
- Assume a boxing stance by keeping your knees slightly bent, shoulders relaxed, and fists clenched.
- Start with a jab by extending your lead arm forward, rotating your wrist to face down, and bringing it back to the starting position.
- Follow up with a cross punch using your rear arm, rotating your hips and shoulders for maximum power.
- Incorporate hooks by bending your elbow and driving your arm in a circular motion to the side, targeting the imaginary opponent's ribs or head.
- Practice defensive moves such as slipping, ducking, or weaving by moving your upper body to avoid imaginary punches.

- Maintain a steady rhythm and fluid motion as you continue to throw a combination of punches and defensive maneuvers.
- Breathe deeply and engage your core muscles throughout the exercise.
- Perform shadow boxing for a duration that suits your fitness level, gradually increasing the intensity and duration over time.

Shadow boxing offers a great cardiovascular workout, helps improve coordination, and can enhance upper body strength. It's important to focus on proper technique and form to maximize the benefits and minimize the risk of injury.

Chair Running

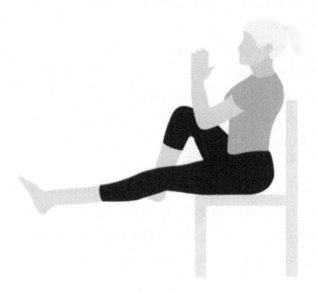

- Sit straight in your chair with both legs extended. Keep your toes pointed and your arms bent at your sides.
- Tighten your abs and lightly touch your shoulder blades to the back of the chair.
- Bend your right knee into your chest and twist the torso towards the knee.
- Your right elbow swings backward while your left one swings forward.
- They change directions as you switch to the left leg.
- Continue alternating sides, bending the knees, twisting the torso, and swinging the elbows
- Aim to perform 25–30 reps in total.
- Focus on engaging your arms, legs, and abs throughout the exercise.

- Maintain a steady pace and rhythm as you perform the movements.
- Remember to breathe steadily and listen to your body's limits.

This exercise provides an enjoyable and effective cardio workout, all while seated.

AGE IS JUST A NUMBER

Robert Marchand, a French cyclist, achieved remarkable athletic feats in his later years. Researchers from the University of Burgundy in Dijon studied elite athletes and found that Marchand, the world record holder in 1-hour track cycling for his age group, stood out as the top athlete over 100 years old.

In his record-breaking attempt, Marchand covered a distance of 26.93 kilometers in one hour, which was 50.6% slower than Bradley Wiggins, the current world record holder. To put this in perspective, another athlete, Donald Pellmann, competing in the 100-meter race for the 100 to 104 age group, finished with a time of 26.99 seconds, a 64.5% decrease compared to Usain Bolt's world record.

Typically, athletic performance starts to decline around the age of 35 to 40, with a decrease of about 10% to 15% per decade. However, Marchand has defied this trend by experiencing a much slower decline of less than 8% per decade for over 60 years.

Born in 1911 in Amiens, France, Marchand began cycling at the age of 14 but had to take a break during his working career. He resumed cycling at the age of 67 and, at 89 years old, completed a grueling 600-kilometer race from Bordeaux to Paris in 36 hours. Marchand's enduring passion and exceptional performance in cycling serve as an inspiration to athletes of all ages (Cycling Today, 2016).

5

CORE EXERCISES

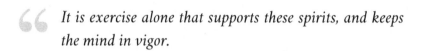 *It is exercise alone that supports these spirits, and keeps the mind in vigor.*

— CICERO

Lean Back

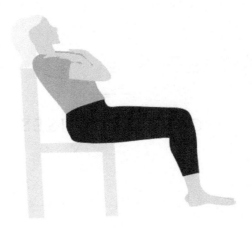

Here are the steps to follow for Chair Seated Crunch:

- Sit on the edge of your chair, ensuring that your feet are flat on the ground and positioned slightly apart.
- Cross your arms over your chest, with your palms touching your shoulders.
- Keeping your spinal alignment intact, lean your upper back towards the backrest of the chair.
- When your upper back touches the backrest, return to the starting position. This completes one repetition.
- For an added challenge, perform the movement slowly, allowing yourself to feel the engagement of your core muscles as they resist gravity.

Remember to maintain proper form and listen to your body during the exercise.

Seated Half Role-Backs

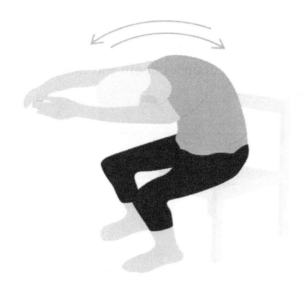

- Sit on your chair with your back straight and feet on the ground, hip-width apart.
- Slowly raise and stretch your arms at chest level.
- Inhale and engage your core muscles by drawing your belly button towards your spine.
- Slowly round your spine, starting from your lower back and continuing up towards your shoulders, as you exhale.
- Keep rolling back until your upper back touches the backrest of the chair.
- Pause for a moment, feeling the stretch and activation in your abdominal muscles.
- Inhale and begin to roll back up, reversing the movement one vertebra at a time until you return to the starting position.

- Repeat the movement for the desired number of repetitions.

Focus on using your core muscles to initiate and control the movement and try to maintain a smooth and controlled motion throughout the exercise.

Seated Forward Roll-Ups

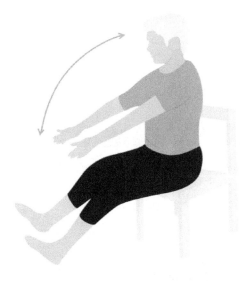

- Sit on the edge of your chair.
- Put your hands over your thighs.
- Inhale deeply, lengthening your spine and sitting tall.
- Exhale as you begin to roll your spine forward, starting from your upper back and moving sequentially through each vertebra.
- Keep rolling forward, allowing your head to come towards your chest and reaching your hands towards your feet.
- Pause in this forward fold position, feeling the stretch in your back and hamstrings.
- Inhale and initiate the movement to roll back up, engaging your core and reversing the motion one vertebra at a time.

- Continue rolling up until you return to the upright seated position with a tall and extended spine.
- Repeat the movement for the desired number of repetitions.

Alternating Oblique Crunch

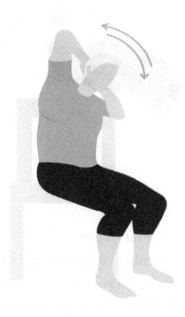

- Sit upright on the edge of a chair with your feet planted firmly on the ground and hip-width apart.
- Place your hands lightly behind your head, with your elbows pointed out to the sides.
- Engage your core by drawing your belly button towards your spine.
- Lift your right foot slightly off the ground, keeping your knee bent.
- As you exhale, bring your right elbow towards your right knee.

- Contract your oblique muscles on the right side as you perform the crunch.
- Breathe in while you go back to the starting position. Repeat the movement on the other side by lifting your left foot and bringing your left elbow towards your left knee.
- Continue alternating sides, performing controlled and deliberate crunches.

If you have any discomfort or pain, modify the range of motion or consult with a healthcare professional.

Alternating Rope Pull

- Begin the exercise by pulling your right hand down towards your right hip as if you are pulling the rope.
- At the same time, extend your left arm up and overhead as if reaching for the sky.
- Hold an imaginary rope with both hands as if you are pulling it down from above your head.
- Focus on squeezing your right shoulder blade and engaging your right side oblique muscles as you perform the pulling motion.
- Return to the starting position and repeat the movement on the other side.

Maintain proper posture throughout the exercise, keeping your spine aligned and your shoulders relaxed.

Twist

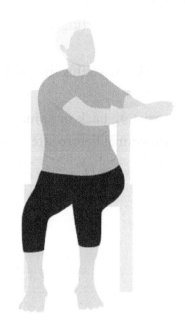

- Sit upright, legs hip-width apart.
- Place your hands on your hips or hold onto the sides of the chair for support.
- Engage your core muscles by drawing your belly button towards your spine.
- Take a deep breath in and lengthen your spine, sitting tall.
- Exhale and slowly begin to twist your torso to the right with your hand in the air following your movements.
- Rotate from your waist, allowing your upper body to follow the movement.
- Keep your hips facing forward and grounded on the chair.

- Hold the twist for a few seconds, feeling the gentle stretch in your oblique muscles.
- Inhale and return to the starting position, sitting upright.
- Exhale and repeat the twist, this time to the left side.

If you have any pre-existing back or spinal conditions, consult with a healthcare professional before attempting this exercise.

Alternating Cross Body Crunch

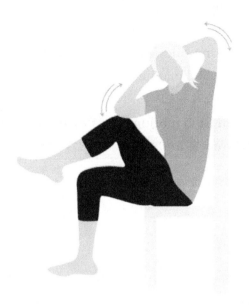

- Sit on the edge of a chair with your feet on the floor and knees bent.
- Position your hands at the back of your head, with your elbows pointing outward.
- Engage your core muscles by drawing your belly button towards your spine.
- Exhale and lift your right knee up towards your chest while simultaneously bringing your left elbow across your body to meet your knee.
- Contract your abdominal muscles as you perform the crunch.
- Inhale and slowly lower your right leg back to the starting position while returning your left elbow to the starting position.

- Repeat the movement on the other side by lifting your left knee and bringing your right elbow across your body to meet your knee.
- Continue alternating sides, performing the cross body crunch in a controlled manner.

Aim for a smooth and fluid motion, focusing on the contraction of the abs with each repetition.

Alternating Side Bend

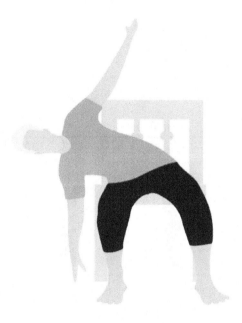

- Sit on a chair with your back straight.
- Place your hands on your hips or let them hang by your sides for support and stability.
- Inhale deeply and engage your core muscles.
- Exhale and slowly lean your upper body to one side, reaching down towards the floor with your hand.
- Keep your spine long and avoid hunching your shoulders.
- Hold the stretch for a few seconds, feeling the stretch on the opposite side of your body.
- Inhale and return to the upright position.
- Repeat the movement on the other side by leaning towards the opposite side and reaching down towards the floor with your hand.

Aim to reach as far as you comfortably can without straining or causing discomfort.

Touch The Floor

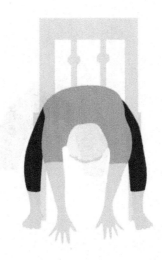

- Sit on a chair with your back straight.
- Place your hands on your thighs or grasp the sides of the chair for support.
- Take a deep breath in and engage your core muscles by drawing your belly button towards your spine.
- As you exhale, gradually tilt forward from your hips, extending your hands towards the floor.
- Maintain a straight back and avoid rounding your shoulders as you reach downward.
- Go as far as your flexibility allows, aiming to touch the floor with your fingertips or palms.
- Hold the stretch for a few seconds, feeling the stretch in your hamstrings and lower back.
- Inhale and slowly return to the upright sitting position.

- Repeat the movement for a desired number of repetitions or as per your comfort level.

Alternating Extended Leg Lift

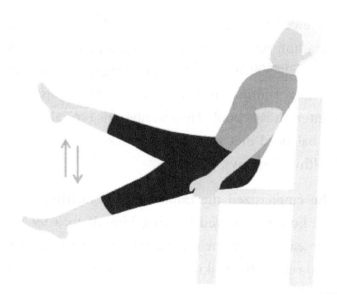

- Sit upright on a chair with your feet flat on the floor and your hands resting on the sides of the chair.
- Engage your core muscles by drawing your belly button towards your spine.
- Extend both legs straight out in front of you, keeping them parallel to the floor. Point your toes forward.
- Raise your right leg slowly and hold it for a few seconds, feeling the tension in your leg muscles.
- Lower your right leg to its initial position. Repeat the same movement with your left leg.
- Continue alternating between your right and left leg.

Aim to maintain a controlled and steady pace throughout the exercise.

AGE IS JUST A NUMBER

Gail Bell interviewed Eugene "Oggie" Winters (who was 62 at the time), a marathon runner who aimed to complete his 475th marathon and reach 500 within the year. Oggie was glad to share his morning routine, including checking emails and engaging in banter on Facebook. He describes his typical meals, emphasizing a balanced diet with salads, chicken or beef, and avoiding unhealthy takeaways.

Additionally, he emphasized the importance of nutrition. He also mentioned how he enjoyed treating himself to a 99 ice cream cone after each marathon. Overall, he doesn't take health supplements and relaxes by walking on Portstewart Strand and gardening (Bell, 2019).

6

STRENGTH TRAINING

 The best day to start exercising is today. Tomorrow can turn into weeks, months or years.

— MARK DILWORTH

STRENGTH TRAINING FOR UPPER BODY

The following upper body exercises can be used with dumbbells, water bottles, or without any weights:

Shoulder Rolls

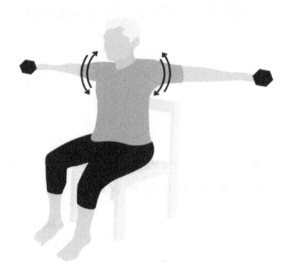

- Sit upright on a chair with your feet on the ground and your hands resting on your thighs.
- Relax your shoulders and take a deep breath in.
- Roll your shoulders using a circular motion.
- Continue the circular motion, gradually increasing the size of the circles. Feel the stretch and tension release in your shoulder muscles.
- After a few repetitions, reverse the direction and roll your shoulders backward, bringing them up and back in a circular motion.

- Repeat the backward shoulder rolls for several repetitions, allowing your shoulder blades to move freely.

Perform shoulder rolls for a desired number of repetitions or until you feel relief and increased mobility in your shoulders.

Chest Press

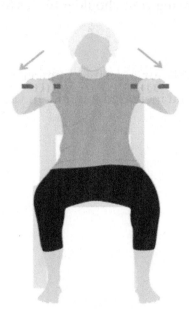

- Sit upright on the edge of a chair.
- Hold dumbbells with your palms facing forward. If you don't have dumbbells, you can use water bottles or any other weighted objects.
- Bend your elbows and bring your arms up to shoulder level, forming a 90-degree angle with your elbows.
- Exhale and push the dumbbells forward, extending your arms straight in front of you. Your palms should face down at this point.
- Hold the extended position for a brief moment, focusing on squeezing your chest muscles.
- Inhale and slowly bring the dumbbells back to the starting position, maintaining control and resistance.

- Repeat the movement for the desired number of repetitions, usually 8–12 reps.

Start with lighter weights and gradually increase the resistance as you become more comfortable and stronger.

Shoulder Press

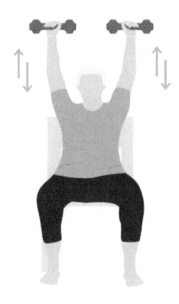

- Sit upright on a chair.
- Hold your dumbbells, palms facing forward, and the weights positioned at shoulder level.
- Engage your core muscles and maintain a neutral spine throughout the exercise.
- Exhale and push the dumbbells upward, extending your arms fully overhead. Keep your palms facing forward as you press the weights.

- Pause briefly at the top of the movement, focusing on contracting your shoulder muscles.
- While breathing in, gradually lower your dumbbells to their initial position.
- Repeat the movement for the desired number of repetitions, typically 8–12 reps.
- Remember to breathe naturally and avoid holding your breath.

Seated Dumbell Row

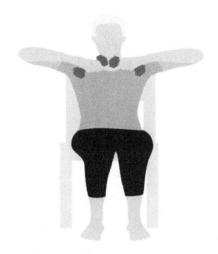

- Sit on a chair with your back straight.
- Hold your dumbbells.
- Your arms should hang down by your sides, palms facing inwards.
- Engage your core muscles and maintain a neutral spine throughout the exercise.
- Lean forward slightly from the hips, keeping your back straight and chest lifted.
- Exhale and slowly lift the dumbbells towards your torso, bending your elbows and squeezing your shoulder blades together. Keep your elbows close to your body as you lift the weights.
- Pause briefly at the top of the movement, focusing on contracting your back muscles.
- Inhale and lower the dumbbells back to the starting position with control, fully extending your arms.

- Repeat the movement for the desired number of repetitions, typically 8–12 reps.

This exercise targets the muscles of the upper back, including the rhomboids, lats, and rear deltoids.

Palm-Up Wrist Curls

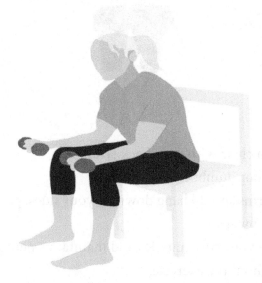

- Sit on a chair with your feet flat on the ground and your knees bent at a 90-degree angle.
- Hold dumbbells or weighted objects in each hand, with your palm facing up. Rest your forearms on your thigh or the edge of the chair, allowing your hands to hang over the edge.
- Your wrists should be in a neutral position.
- Slowly breathe out and curl your wrists upward, lifting the weight as high as possible while keeping your forearms stationary.

- Pause briefly at the top of the movement, focusing on squeezing your wrist flexors.
- Slowly lower the weight as you breathe out.
- As you do so, allow your wrists to extend.
- Repeat the movement for the desired number of repetitions, typically 8–12 reps.

If you experience any pain or discomfort, stop the exercise and consult with a healthcare professional.

Lateral Raise

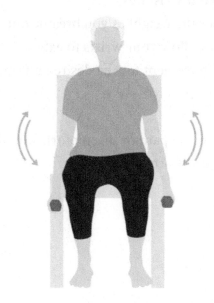

- Sit on a chair, keep your back straight, and engage your core muscles.
- Hold a dumbbell or a weighted object in each hand, with your palms facing your body.
- Exhale and slowly raise both arms out to the sides, away from your body. Keep your elbows slightly bent and maintain control throughout the movement.
- Continue lifting your arms until they reach shoulder level or slightly below while keeping your wrists in a neutral position.
- Inhale and slowly lower your arms back down to the starting position, returning to the resting position with control.
- Repeat the movement for the desired number of repetitions, typically 8–12 reps.

This exercise targets the deltoid muscles in the shoulders, specifically the lateral (middle) deltoids.

Bicep Curls

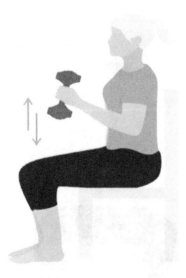

- Sit on a chair with your feet flat on the ground, knees bent at a 90-degree angle, and back straight.
- Hold a dumbbell or a weighted object in each hand, with your palms facing forward.
- Keep your elbows close to your body and exhale as you slowly lift the weights toward your shoulders.
- Keep your wrists straight, and avoid using momentum to swing the weights upward. Focus on using your bicep muscles to perform the movement.
- Inhale and slowly lower the weights back down to the starting position, maintaining control throughout the movement.

- Repeat the exercise for the desired number of repetitions, typically 8–12 reps.

This exercise helps to strengthen and tone the biceps.

Tricep Curls

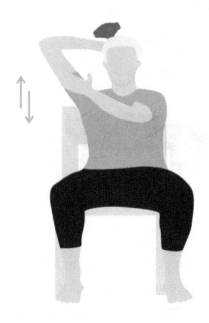

- Sit on a chair with your feet flat on the ground and back straight.
- Hold a dumbbell or a weighted object in one hand, with your palm facing inwards and your arm extended straight up.
- Bend your elbow and lower the weight behind your head, keeping your upper arm stationary and close to your head.

- Pause briefly at the bottom of the movement, feeling the stretch in your triceps.
- Exhale and straighten your arm to return to the starting position without locking your elbow.
- Repeat the exercise for the desired number of repetitions on one arm before switching to the other arm.

This exercise targets the muscles in the back of your upper arms, specifically the triceps brachii. It also helps to strengthen and tone the triceps.

STRENGTH TRAINING FOR LOWER BODY

Heel Slides

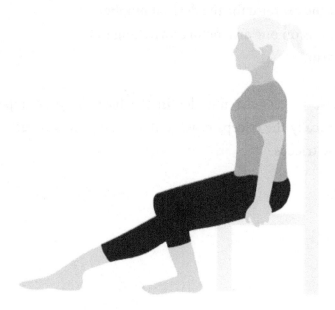

- Sit on a chair with your back straight and feet flat on the floor.
- Slide one heel forward along the floor, straightening your knee as much as possible.
- Slowly return your heel back to the starting position.
- Repeat the movement with the other leg.
- Continue alternating heel slides for the desired number of repetitions.

Heel slides target the muscles of the lower body, particularly the quadriceps.

Leg Kicks

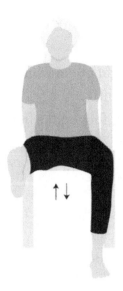

- Sit on a chair with your back straight and feet flat on the floor.
- Keep your knee bent as you extend one leg in front of you.
- Kick your leg forward, aiming to straighten it as much as possible.
- Slowly put your leg down to its initial position.
- Repeat the exercise using your other leg.
- Continue alternating leg kicks for the desired number of repetitions.

Leg kicks can help strengthen and tone the muscles of the legs, improve balance, and increase flexibility.

Single-Leg Calf Raises

- Sit on the edge of a chair with your back straight and feet flat on the floor.
- Extend one leg straight out in front of you, keeping your knee slightly bent.
- Place the ball of your foot on the floor while keeping your heel lifted.
- Engage your calf muscle and slowly raise your heel as high as possible.
- Hold the raised position for a brief moment, focusing on contracting your calf muscle.
- Lower your heel back down to the starting position in a controlled manner.
- Repeat the movement for the desired number of repetitions.
- Switch legs and repeat the exercise on the opposite side.

Single-leg calf raises target the calf muscles in your lower legs. They help to strengthen and tone your calves while improving balance and stability.

Sit-to-Stands

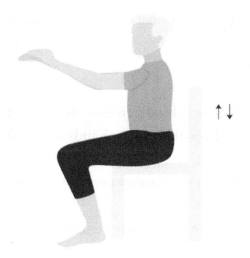

- Sit by the chair edge.
- Keep your back straight and engage your core muscles.
- Lift your hands to your chest with one palm on top of the other, or cross them over your chest.
- Lean slightly forward and shift your weight onto your feet.
- Slowly stand up, pushing through your heels and keeping your knees aligned with your toes.
- Fully extend your hips and straighten your legs as you rise to a standing position.
- Pause for a moment at the top, maintaining balance and stability.
- Return to the seated position as you gently bend your hips and knees.
- Control the descent and aim to lightly touch the chair before repeating the movement.

This exercise strengthens the lower body, particularly the legs and glutes. It mimics the motion of standing up from a seated position, making it a functional exercise for everyday activities.

Modified Squat

- Begin by standing behind a chair with your feet shoulder-width apart. Put your hands on the chair for support if needed.
- Position your feet so that they are slightly turned outwards.
- Slowly lower your body down, bending at the hips and knees.
- Keep your weight in your heels as you lower yourself down as if you are sitting back in the chair.
- Pause for a moment in the seated position, and then push through your heels to rise back up to the starting position.
- Fully extend your hips and knees as you stand up. Repeat the movement for the desired number of repetitions.

Make sure to keep your knees aligned with your toes and avoid letting them collapse inward.

Hip Abduction

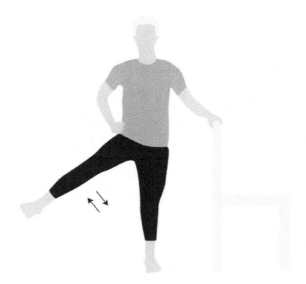

- Stand tall next to a chair with your feet hip-width apart.
- Hold onto the back of the chair for support and stability.
- Engage your core muscles to maintain proper posture throughout the exercise.
- Shift your weight onto one leg while keeping a slight bend in your knees.
- Slowly lift your other leg out to the side as high as possible while keeping your toes pointed forward.
- Focus on using the muscles of your outer thigh to lift your leg rather than relying on momentum.
- Pause briefly at the top of the movement, feeling the contraction in your outer thigh.
- Gradually lower your leg.

- Repeat the movement for the desired number of repetitions on one side before switching to the other leg.

Hip abduction targets the muscles of the outer thighs and hips. It also helps strengthen the hip muscles and improve stability.

Knee Extension

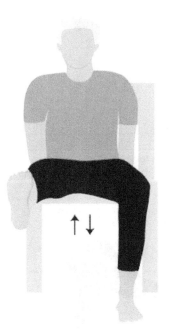

- Sit on a chair with your back straight and feet flat on the floor.
- Place your hands on the sides of the chair for stability.
- Extend one leg out in front of you, keeping your knee straight and your foot flexed.
- Hold the extended position for a brief moment, feeling the contraction in your quadriceps muscles.
- Gently return your leg to the initial position, lowering it down slowly.
- Repeat the movement with the other leg.
- Continue alternating legs for the desired number of repetitions.

This exercise targets the quadriceps muscles in the front of the thigh. It is particularly useful for individuals who may have difficulty performing standing exercises or those recovering from knee injuries.

Glute Kick Back

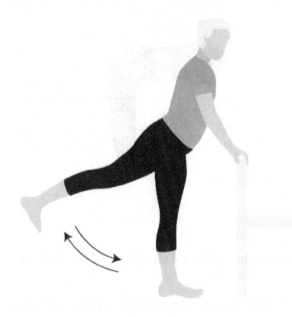

- Stand behind a chair with your feet hip-width apart and your hands lightly resting on the back of the chair for support.
- Shift your weight onto one leg while keeping a slight bend in your supporting leg.
- Slowly lift your other leg behind you, focusing on squeezing your glute muscles to lift the leg.
- Continue lifting your leg until it is parallel to the floor or until you feel a contraction in your glutes.

- Pause for a moment at the top of the movement, emphasizing the squeeze in your glute muscles.
- Gently return your leg to the initial position, lowering it down slowly.
- Repeat the movement on the same leg for the desired number of repetitions.
- Switch legs and perform the exercise on the other side.

This is a great exercise for targeting and strengthening the gluteal muscles, particularly the gluteus maximus. It helps to improve hip stability, enhance lower body strength, and shape the buttocks.

AGE IS JUST A NUMBER

Eighty-two-year-old Willie Murphy, an award-winning female bodybuilder, demonstrated her bravery when she fought off a home intruder in Rochester, New York. Upon hearing pounding on her front door, Murphy wisely called the police instead of letting the intruder inside, despite his pleas for help.

Murphy's impressive physical abilities (including her strength in deadlifting 225 pounds and mastering challenging exercises) gave her a clear advantage over the intruder. The man had deceived Murphy by falsely claiming to be shot and in need of assistance to gain entry, but he soon realized he had underestimated her strength.

In her living room, Murphy courageously defended herself by delivering powerful blows to the intruder. Determined to protect herself, she fought back with all her might. The intruder was no match for her and had to be taken to the hospital for treatment.

Remarkably, Murphy emerged from the encounter unharmed. The responding police officers were so impressed with her courage and strength that they requested to take selfies with her.

Willie Murphy's remarkable story highlights not only her physical prowess but also her resilience and refusal to be a victim. She serves as an inspiration and a powerful reminder that age should never hinder strength and the ability to defend oneself.

7

20-MINUTE ROUTINES

 All progress takes place outside the comfort zone.

— MICHAEL JOHN BOBAK

The following exercise routines are my personal recommendations. It's crucial to note that these routines may need to be modified to suit an individual's health and fitness level. The number of repetitions and duration can be adjusted accordingly. Additionally, it's essential to allocate time for a proper cool down, which may include stretching or other appropriate activities (you can use warm-up exercises at a slower pace for a cool down). Taking these factors into consideration will help ensure a safe and effective exercise session.

ROUTINE #1: ALL ABOUT STRETCHING/YOGA

Warm-Up (4 minutes)

- Neck Releasing Pose (chapter 3): 2–4 reps, 1 minute
- Cow Face Pose (chapter 3): 2-4 reps, 1 minute
- Seated Mountain (chapter 3): 2-4 reps, 1 minute
- Shoulder Opener (chapter 3): 2-4 reps, 1 minute

Exercises (16 minutes)

- Cat and Cow Stretch (chapter 3): 4-8 reps, 2 minutes
- Chair Spinal Twist (chapter 3): 4-8 reps, 2 minutes
- Side Bend (chapter 3): 4-8 reps, 2 minutes
- Chair Eagle—Garudasana (chapter 3): 4-8 reps, 2 minutes
- Overhead Stretch (chapter 3): 4-8 reps, 2 minutes
- Flex and Stretch (chapter 3): 4-8 reps, 2 minutes
- Chair Extended Side Angle (chapter 3): 4-8 reps, 2 minutes
- Seated Forward Bend (chapter 3): 4-8 reps, 2 minutes

Work your way up to adding:

- Chair Warrior I—Virabhadrasana I (chapter 3)
- Chair Warrior II—Virabhadrasana II (chapter 3)
- Reverse Warrior (chapter 3)
- Half-splits pose with a chair (chapter 3)

ROUTINE #2: ARM DAY

Warm-Up (4 minutes):

- Shoulder Opener (chapter 3): 4–8 reps, 1 minute
- Tricep Shoulder Stretch (chapter 3): 4-8 reps, 1 minute
- Head Circle (chapter 3): 4–8 reps, 1 minute
- Arm Circle (chapter 4): 4–8 reps, 1 minute

Exercises: With Dumbbells (16 minutes)

- Shoulder Rolls (chapter 6): 8–16 reps, 2 minutes
- Chest Press (chapter 6): 8–16 reps, 2 minutes
- Shoulder Press (chapter 6): 8–16 reps, 2 minutes
- Seated Dumbbell Row (chapter 6): 8–16 reps, 2 minutes
- Palm-up Wrist Curls (chapter 6): 8–16 reps, 2 minutes
- Lateral Raise (chapter 6): 8–16 reps, 2 minutes
- Bicep Curls (chapter 6): 8–16 reps, 2 minutes
- Tricep Curls (chapter 6): 8–16 reps, 2 minutes

ROUTINE #3: LEG DAY

Warm-Up (4 minutes):

- Heel Raise (chapter 3): 4-8 reps, 1 minute
- Knee Lift (chapter 4): 4-8 reps, 1 minute
- Chair Running (chapter 4): 1 minute
- Chair Eagle (chapter 3): 4-8 reps, 1 minute

Exercises (16 minutes):

- Heel Slides (chapter 6): 8–16 reps, 2 minutes
- Single-Leg Calf Raises (chapter 6): 8–16 reps, 2 minutes
- Single Leg Forward Bend (chapter 3): 8–16 reps, 2 minutes
- Sit-to-Stand (chapter 6): 8–16 reps, 2 minutes
- Modified Squats (chapter 6): 8–16 reps, 2 minutes
- Hip-Abduction (chapter 6): 8–16 reps, 2 minutes
- Glute Kick Back (chapter 6): 8–16 reps, 2 minutes
- Leg Kicks (chapter 6): 8-16 reps, 2 minutes

ROUTINE #4: CORE AND CARDIO DAY

Warm-Up (4 minutes):

- Overhead Stretch (chapter 3): 8-16 reps, 1 minute
- Arm Cross (chapter 4): 8-16 reps, 1 minute
- Heel Raise (chapter 3): 8-16 reps, 1 minute
- Knee Lift (chapter 4): 8-16 reps, 1 minute

Exercises (16 minutes)

Cardio (8 minutes)

- Alternating Side Reach High (chapter 4): 8–16 reps, 1 minute
- Alternating Side Reach Low (chapter 4): 8–16 reps, 1 minute

- Alternating Cross Body Knee Reach (chapter 4): 8–16 reps, 1 minute
- Alternating Cross Body Toe Touch (chapter 4): 8–16 reps, 1 minute
- Seated Jacks (chapter 4): 8–16 reps, 1 minute
- Skater Switch (chapter 4): 8–16 reps, 1 minute
- Shadow Boxing (Chapter 4): 1 minute
- Chair Running (chapter 4): 1 minute

Core (8 minutes)

- Lean Back (chapter 5): 8–16 reps, 1 minute
- Twist (chapter 5): 8–16 reps, 1 minute
- Touch the Floor (chapter 5): 8–16 reps, 1 minute
- Seated Forward Roll-ups (chapter 5): 8–16 reps, 1 minute
- Seated Forward Role-backs (chapter 5): 8–16 reps, 1 minute
- Alternating Oblique Crunch (chapter 5): 8–16 reps, 1 minute
- Alternating Extended Leg Lift (chapter 5): 8–16 reps, 1 minute
- Alternating Side Bend (chapter 5): 8–16 reps, 1 minute

Remember, you can modify/add onto any of the above routines to keep up with their latest advancements or enhance your workout routines.

AGE IS JUST A NUMBER

Charles Eugster, a 96-year-old bodybuilder and sprinter, challenged the notion of retirement, saying that staying active and productive is crucial for healthy aging. Eugster emphasized the importance of older individuals making meaningful contributions to society rather than being forced into retirement.

Eugster didn't start weight training until the age of 87 and began running at 95. He promoted the idea that it's never too late to get in shape and build muscle, as older adults tend to lose muscle mass with age. He also advised employing high-intensity interval training, allowing for proper recovery time, maintaining a healthy waistline, trying new sports or activities, and using protein and vitamin D supplements to support muscle growth.

Eugster said his ultimate goal was to change society's perception of aging, encouraging older adults to embrace a fulfilling and active lifestyle. He believes that it's possible to rebuild and improve one's body at any age and that life can become even more fulfilling as we grow older (Stump, 2016).

8

EXERCISE LOGBOOK

Here's a sample workout log to help you track your exercises:

Date:

Warm-up:

- Gentle neck rotations: ___repetitions
- Shoulder rolls: ___ repetitions
- Arm circles: ___ repetitions
- March in place: ___ minutes

Exercise 1: Chair Squats

- Sets: ___ Reps: ___ Notes: _____

Exercise 2: Seated Leg Extensions

- Sets: ___ Reps: ___ Notes: _____

Exercise 3: Chair Dips

- Sets: ___ Reps: ___ Notes: _____

Exercise 4: Seated Arm Curls

- Sets: ___ Reps: ___ Notes: _____

Exercise 5: Leg Raises

- Sets: ___ Reps: ___ Notes: _____

Exercise 6: Seated Side Bends

- Sets: ___ Reps: ___ Notes: _____

Exercise 7: Seated Shoulder Press

- Sets: ___ Reps: ___ Notes: _____

Exercise 8: Seated Chest Press

- Sets: ___ Reps: ___ Notes: _____

Exercise 9: Seated Tricep Extensions

- Sets: ___ Reps: ___ Notes: _____

Exercise 10: Seated Core Twists

- Sets: ___ Reps: ___ Notes: _____

Cool Down:

- Gentle seated forward bend: ___ repetitions
- Shoulder and upper back stretches: ___ repetitions
- Deep breathing and relaxation: ___ minutes

Notes/Comments: _____

Use this workout log to track your progress and adjust the sets, reps, and intensity as needed. Make sure to perform each exercise with proper form and listen to your body. Gradually increase the number of sets, reps, or difficulty levels as you become more comfortable and stronger.

Remember, always consult with your healthcare provider before starting any new exercise program, especially if you have any underlying health conditions.

Enjoy your chair exercises, and have a wonderful workout!

CONCLUSION

In the journey of life, reaching our senior years should be celebrated as a testament to the wisdom and experiences we have gained. However, it's no secret that the aging process brings certain challenges, including a decline in physical strength and mobility. Fortunately, the power to reclaim our vitality and live life to the fullest lies within our grasp. Through the practice of low-impact and gentle chair exercises, seniors can embark on a transformative path towards improved health, enhanced well-being, and a renewed sense of joy.

In this book, we have explored a comprehensive range of chair exercises specifically designed for seniors, taking into account the unique needs and abilities of older adults. We have seen how these exercises can be tailored to accommodate various fitness levels, ensuring that everyone can participate and benefit from this form of physical activity. The beauty of chair exercises lies not only in their accessibility but also in their effectiveness in promoting strength, flexibility, balance, and overall fitness.

One of the greatest advantages of chair exercises is their low-impact nature, making them gentle on the joints and reducing the risk of injury. By eliminating the need for complex equipment or excessive strain on the body, these exercises provide a safe and supportive environment for seniors to engage in physical activity. Whether recovering from an injury, managing chronic conditions, or simply seeking to maintain a healthy lifestyle, chair exercises offer an ideal solution for older adults to stay active and vibrant.

Throughout this book, we have demonstrated the diverse array of exercises that can be performed while seated, showcasing the versatility and creativity that can be incorporated into a senior's fitness routine. From gentle stretches and range of motion exercises to targeted strength training and cardiovascular movements, there is an exercise for every individual, regardless of their physical limitations or previous fitness experience. Chair exercises can be modified and adapted to meet the specific needs of each senior, ensuring a personalized approach to fitness.

Beyond the physical benefits, engaging in regular chair exercises has far-reaching effects on mental and emotional well-being. Physical activity stimulates the release of endorphins, often referred to as "feel-good" hormones, which can elevate mood, reduce stress, and improve overall mental clarity. Chair exercises provide an opportunity for seniors to connect with their bodies, cultivate mindfulness, and experience a sense of accomplishment. The resulting boost in self-confidence and self-esteem can have a profound impact on the overall quality of life.

Moreover, chair exercises have the power to foster a sense of community and social connection among seniors. Engaging in group exercise classes or sharing workout routines with friends and loved ones can create a supportive network of like-minded individuals who encourage and inspire each other on their wellness journey. The camaraderie that develops through these shared experiences fosters a sense of belonging and combats feelings of isolation that may accompany aging.

As we conclude our exploration of low-impact and gentle chair exercises for seniors, it's important to recognize that the journey to improved health and vitality is ongoing. Consistency and dedication are key to reaping the full benefits of regular physical activity. By incorporating chair exercises into a daily routine, you can gradually build strength, increase flexibility, and improve overall fitness levels. It's a journey that requires patience, perseverance, and an unwavering belief in the transformative power of movement.

In closing, I encourage every senior who has read this book to embrace the journey toward a healthier, more active life. Let these chair exercises become a cornerstone of your wellness routine, empowering you to age gracefully and embrace your full potential. Remember, it's never too late to embark on a path of self-care and well-being. With each movement, you are reclaiming your vitality, nurturing your body, and celebrating the joy of living life to the fullest.

REFERENCES

Abbate, E. (2022, April 25). *Here's what a perfectly balanced weekly workout schedule looks like.* Shape. https://www.shape.com/fitness/training-plans/perfectly-balanced-week-workouts

A.I.M. Fitness-Activities in Motion. (2019, November 12). *Cardio chair exercises for seniors* [Video]. Youtube. https://www.youtube.com/watch?v=0pxvqa3_lMI

Ambrose, S. (n.d.). *How to do: Sitting flutter kicks.* Skimble. https://www.skimble.com/exercises/15174-sitting-flutter-kicks-how-to-do-exercise

Arm workouts for seniors and the elderly. (n.d.). Eldergym. https://eldergym.com/arm-workouts/

Bedosky, L. (2022, April 2). *The best core exercises for seniors.* Get Healthy U. https://gethealthyu.com/best-core-exercises-for-seniors/

Bell, G. (2019, May 1). *A 99 at the finish line keeps 62-year-old Oggie on the road to 500 marathons.* The Irish News. https://www.irishnews.com/lifestyle/2019/05/01/news/a-99-at-the-finish-line-keeps-62-year-old-oggie-on-the-road-to-500-marathons-1608392/

Better Health Channel. (n.d.-a). *Exercise safety.* https://www.betterhealth.vic.gov.au/health/healthyliving/exercise-safety#exercise-safety-advice

Better Health Channel. (n.d.-b). *Physical activity—setting yourself goals.* https://www.betterhealth.vic.gov.au/health/healthyliving/physical-activity-setting-yourself-goals

Bhardwaj, N. (2021, June 15). *Try this 11-minute seated cardio to lose 2 kilos in 30 days.* Healthshots. https://www.healthshots.com/fitness/weight-loss/try-this-11-minute-seated-cardio-to-lose-2-kilos-in-30-days/

Bicep curls exercise. (n.d.). More Life Health. https://morelifehealth.com/bicep-curls

Biswas, C. (2023, June 16). *15 easy and effective chair exercises for seniors.* StyleCraze. https://www.stylecraze.com/articles/chair-exercises-for-seniors/

Blick, K. (2017, December 14). *Energize your workday with upper-body chair yoga.* Allina Health. https://www.allinahealth.org/healthysetgo/move/energize-your-workday-with-upperbody-chair-yoga

Burkhart, L. (2019, August 8). *Shoulder and neck chair yoga that you can do anywhere, anytime.* Wysefit. https://wysefit.com/blog/shoulder-and-neck-chair-yoga-that-you-can-do-anywhere-anytime/

CareLink. (2021, September 21). *Benefits of chair exercises for seniors.* https://www.carelink.org/benefits-of-chair-exercises-for-seniors/

Centers for Disease Control and Prevention. (2017). *Risk factors for falls.* https://www.cdc.gov/steadi/pdf/STEADI-FactSheet-RiskFactors-508.pdf

Centers for Disease Control and Prevention. (2023, March 24). *Keep on your feet—preventing older adult falls.* https://www.cdc.gov/injury/features/older-adult-falls/index.html

Centers for Disease Control and Prevention. (n.d.). *How much physical activity do older adults need?* https://www.cdc.gov/physicalactivity/basics/older_adults/index.htm

Cerqua, P. & Bobinger, A. (2023, May 4). *How to motivate yourself to work out.* WikiHow. https://www.wikihow.com/Motivate-Yourself-to-Work-Out

Chair yoga poses. (n.d.). Tumme.com. https://www.tummee.com/yoga-poses/chair-yoga-poses

Courtney, S. (2018, November 13). *Exercise Of the week: Seated dumbbell row.* Courtney Medical Group. https://courtneymedicalgroupaz.com/2018/11/13/exercise-of-the-week-seated/

Cronkleton, E. (2020, May 29). *12 yoga poses for neck pain.* Healthline. https://www.healthline.com/health/yoga-for-neck-pain#poses

Cycling Today. (2016, November 12). *104-year-old cyclist named world's greatest centenarian athlete.* https://cycling.today/104-year-old-cyclist-named-worlds-greatest-centenarian-athlete/

Cyprus, S. (2023, June 8). *What are chair exercises?* Wisegeek. https://www.wise-geek.com/what-are-chair-exercises.htm

DuBois, M. (2019, June 19). *103-year-old runner Julia "Hurricane" Hawkins breaks new record.* CBS News. https://www.cbsnews.com/news/julia-hurricane-hawkins-runner-breaks-new-record-2019-06-19/

8 best core exercises for seniors. (n.d.). Lifeline. https://www.lifeline.ca/en/resources/core-exercises-for-seniors/

Elbow exercises for seniors and the elderly. (n.d.). Eldergym. https://eldergym.com/elbow-exercises/

Evers, C. (2022, May 1). *How to do standing calf raises: Proper form, variations, and common mistakes.* Verywell Fit. https://www.verywellfit.com/how-to-do-calf-raises-4801090

Fairview ADC. (2019, February 25). *The benefits of chair aerobics for older adults.* Fairview Adult Day Care Center. https://fairviewadc.com/rehabilitation/chair-aerobics-benefits-older-adults/

Familydoctor.org. (2022, May). *Exercise and seniors.* https://familydoctor.org/exercise-seniors/

Fancy, L. (2020, March 20). *6 ways for seniors to stay safe while exercising.* Home Care Assistance. https://www.homecareassistancewinnipeg.ca/how-can-aging-adults-exercise-safely/

Frey, M. (2022, July 28). *How to do a triceps extension: Proper form, variations, and common mistakes.* Verywell Fit. https://www.verywellfit.com/how-to-do-a-triceps-extension-techniques-benefits-variations-5082227

Galantino, M. L., Green, L., DeCesari, J. A., Mackain, N. A., Rinaldi, S. M., Stevens, M. E., Wurst, V. R., Marsico, R., Nell, M., & Mao, J. J. (2012). Safety and feasibility of modified chair-yoga on functional outcome among elderly at risk for falls. *International Journal of Yoga, 5*(2), 146 https://www.ncbi.nlm.nih.gov/pmc/articles/PMC3410195/

Gonzalez, M. (n.d.). *Chair yoga exercises for the feet and toes.* Little Flower Yoga. https://www.littlefloweryoga.com/blog/chair-yoga-exercises-for-the-feet-and-toes

Hanna, S., & Norman, A. (n.d.). *Chair based exercise.* Southern Cambridgeshire Falls Prevention Service. https://laterlifetraining.co.uk/wp-content/uploads/2011/01/Chair-Based-Exercise_Cambridge.pdf

Haworth, J. (2019, November 25). *Female bodybuilder, 82, beats home intruder so badly he had to be taken to hospital.* ABC News. https://abcnews.go.com/US/female-bodybuilder-82-beats-home-intruder-badly-hospital/story?id=67289683

Healthwise Staff. (2022, March 9). *Wrist tendinitis: Exercises.* MyHealth. Alberta.ca https://myhealth.alberta.ca/Health/aftercareinformation/pages/conditions.aspx?hwid=bo1652

Heather. (n.d.). *17 ways to stay motivated to exercise.* Better Living. https://onbetterliving.com/fitness-motivation/

Heger, E. & Wade, G. (2022, February 7). *This personal trainer-approved weekly workout schedule balances strength, cardio, and rest days.* (n.d.). Health. https://www.health.com/fitness/workout-schedule

Hegg, J. (n.d.). *Prevent falls with 5 warning signs of mobility issues in seniors.* DailyCaring. https://dailycaring.com/prevent-falls-with-5-warning-signs-of-mobility-issues-in-seniors/

How to achieve your fitness goals. (n.d.). Maximum Fitness Vacaville. https://www.maximumfitnessvacaville.com/blog/7-steps-how-achieve-common-fitness-goals

HUR USA. (2019, August 6). *4 ways to help seniors tap into lifelong motivation for exercise.* https://hurusa.com/4-ways-to-help-seniors-tap-into-lifelong-motivation-for-exercise/

Immaculate Blog. (2021, April 14). *7 Exercise safety tips for seniors.* Immaculate Home Care. https://immaculatehcs.com/blog/7-exercise-safety-tips-for-seniors/

Improved Health. (2022, April 20). *Seated core strength workout for seniors* [Video]. YouTube. https://www.youtube.com/watch?v=ngGS9NJh_8U

Infographic: Top 10 chair yoga positions for seniors. (n.d.). Senior Lifestyle. https://www.seniorlifestyle.com/resources/blog/infographic-top-10-chair-yoga-positions-for-seniors/

Jaul, E., & Barron, J. (2017). Age-related diseases and clinical and public health implications for the 85 years old and over population. *Frontiers in Public Health, 5.* https://doi.org/10.3389/fpubh.2017.00335

Koenig, R. (2020, February 22). *The world's oldest yoga teacher, Tao Porchon-Lynch, has died at age 101.* Today. https://www.today.com/popculture/tao-porchon-lynch-world-s-oldest-yoga-teacher-dead-101-t174482

Kumar, A. (2019, April 19). *Flo Filion Meiler, an 84-year-old record-breaking pole vaulter, is just getting started.* ESPN. https://www.espn.com/espnw/life-style/story/_/id/26557052/flo-filion-meiler-84-year-old-record-break ing-pole-vaulter-just-getting-started

Kutcher, M. (2018, December 11). *Hip exercises for seniors | Hip stretches for seniors.* More Life Health. https://morelifehealth.com/articles/hip-exer cises-for-seniors

Landgraf, B. (2021, September 14). *How to do cardio while sitting.* Carex. https://carex.com/blogs/resources/how-to-do-cardio-while-sitting

Liliane. (2021, April 26). *50 inspiring senior fitness quotes to keep you moving.* Lo Aids. https://loaids.com/senior-fitness-quotes/

Lindberg, S. (2023, January, 3). *15 chair exercises that will light up your entire body.* SELF. https://www.self.com/gallery/chair-exercises

Live Lean TV Daily Exercises. (2016, October 13). *How to do a seated dumbbell lateral raise | Exercise demonstration video and guide* [Video]. YouTube. https://www.youtube.com/watch?v=djTVHrWCvw8&t=1s

Malmstrom, T. K. & Tait, R. C. (2010.). Chapter 24—Pain assessment and management in older adults. *ScienceDirect, 2.* 647–677. https://doi.org/10. 1016/B978-0-12-374961-1.10024-7

Marchese. G. (2021, April 10). *8 yoga poses to soothe neck pain & tension.* Yoga Journal. https://www.yogajournal.com/poses/anatomy/neck/8-yoga-poses-to-soothe-neck-tension/

May, K. (2020, March 27). *6 common reasons for limited mobility in aging adults.* Home Care Assistance. https://www.homecareassistanceamarillo.com/ what-can-cause-my-elderly-parent-to-have-reduced-mobility/

Mayo Clinic. (2022, November 3). *Aging: What to expect.* https://www. mayoclinic.org/healthy-lifestyle/healthy-aging/in-depth/aging/art-20046070

McCoy, J. (2019, January 3). *How to set realistic fitness goals you'll actually achieve, according to top trainers.* SELF. https://www.self.com/story/how-to-set-realistic-fitness-goals

Mindful Breath. (2020, July 19). *Four chair yoga poses to release tight shoulders, neck and back.* https://mindfulbreath.sg/four-chair-yoga-poses-to-release-tight-shoulders-neck-and-back-mindfulbreath-y/

More Life Health Seniors. (2019, April 10). *Best arms, shoulders & legs exercises for seniors! | Seniors' chair exercises | More life health* [Video]. YouTube. https://www.youtube.com/watch?v=NHwWx2OhRMs

National Council on Aging. (2021, August 30). *The life-changing benefits of exercise after 60.* https://ncoa.org/article/the-life-changing-benefits-of-exercise-after-60

National Council on Aging. (2023, March 13). *Get the facts on falls prevention.* https://ncoa.org/article/get-the-facts-on-falls-prevention

Nera, S. (2021, March 8). *Exercise safety tips for seniors and older adults: Preventing Injury.* Hello Doctor. https://hellodoctor.com.ph/healthy-aging/ exercise-safety-tips-for-seniors/

Nied, J. (2022, October 5). *20 chair exercises for a total-body strength and cardio workout.* Women's Health. https://www.womenshealthmag.com/fitness/ g41252448/best-chair-exercises/

Pahla B, Weight Loss Coach for Women Over 50. (2018, January 8). *Seated sweat | Effective 20 minute no impact all cardio fat burning HIIT workout in a chair* [Video]. YouTube. https://youtu.be/ZmASduS97YY

Pain Theory. (2012, February 11). *Seated hamstring stretch 1* [Video]. YouTube. https://www.youtube.com/watch?v=ykOlGxeEnr0

Pain Theory. (2012, February 11). *Seated hamstring stretch 2* [Video]. YouTube.

https://www.youtube.com/watch?v=kWJQLTIvONY

Paul Eugene. (2019, April 22). *Seated boxing workout—for people with limited mobility | Sit and get fit!* [Video]. YouTube. https://www.youtube.com/watch?v=bTDHO07igD4

Peterson, J. A. (2009). 10 common-sense safety tips for exercise enthusiasts. *ACSM's Health & Fitness Journal, 13*(2), 46. https://doi.org/10.1249/fit.0b013e3181998c64

Petty, M. (2020, August 27). *The body part you really should be working: Your wrists.* Greatist. https://greatist.com/health/how-to-strengthen-wrists#habits-for-healthy-wrists

Pizer, A. (2022, November 4). *10 chair yoga poses you can do at home.* Verywell Fit. https://www.verywellfit.com/chair-yoga-poses-3567189

Power of Positivity. (2020, June 8). *Yogi reveals 10 chair yoga moves for people with knee pain.* https://www.powerofpositivity.com/chair-yoga-seated-poses-for-knee-pain/

Qvortrup, T. (2023, May 2). *The 9 best chair yoga poses you can do at your desk.* yogajala. https://yogajala.com/best-chair-yoga-poses/

Rao, J. (2023, June 6). *5 best chair cardio exercises to burn calories.* StyleCraze. https://www.stylecraze.com/articles/best-chair-cardio-exercises-to-burn-calories/

Reyes, M. (2021, December 5). *Seated spinal twist benefits and how to.* Yoga Rove. https://yogarove.com/seated-spinal-twist-tutorial/

Robeck, I. (2012, December 12). Chronic pain in the elderly: Special challenges. *Practical Pain Management, 12*(2). https://www.practicalpainmanagement.com/pain/chronic-pain-elderly-special-challenges

Robinson, L., Smith, M., & Segal, J. (2023, March 1). *Senior exercise and fitness tips.* HelpGuide.org. https://www.helpguide.org/articles/healthy-living/exercise-and-fitness-as-you-age.htm

Saman. (2020, September 15). *Seated shoulder press harder than standing? why?* Healthy and Happy Life.. https://myservice4all.com/seated-dumbbell-press/#:

Savage, J. (n.d.). *Chair yoga sequence for hips and hamstrings.* Ekhart Yoga. https://www.ekhartyoga.com/articles/practice/chair-yoga-sequence-hips-and-hamstrings

Scalena, M. (n.d.). *7 benefits of daily seated exercise.* Sunshine Centres for Seniors. https://sunshinecentres.com/7-benefits-of-daily-seated-exercise/

Seated cardio boxing workout for seniors and beginners | 20 Min. (n.d.). Senior

Fitness with Meredith. https://www.seniorfitnesswithmeredith.com/seated-cardio-boxing-workout-for-seniors-and-beginners-20-min/

Seated dumbbell exercises for seniors. (2021, October 19). Factory Weights. https://www.factoryweights.co.uk/blogs/news/seated-dumbbell-exercises-for-seniors

Senior Fitness With Meredith. (2020, June 21). Senior fitness—lower body exercises for beginners [Video]. YouTube. https://www.youtube.com/watch?v=Iyn80z-LQNU

Senior Fitness With Meredith. (2022, May 29). The best seated abs and core workout for seniors and beginners / 10min [Video]. YouTube. https://www.youtube.com/watch?v=fLf07p5Q_jY

SeniorShape Fitness. (2020, August 11). Chair cardio workout for seniors & beginners // 30 minute easy exercises at home [Video]. YouTube. https://www.youtube.com/watch?v=yiEX9NPE354&t=9s

Sgargetta, D. (2017, January 12). 20 fitness motivation quotes. Life Fitness. https://www.lifefitness.com.au/20-fitness-motivation-quotes/

Shinners, R. & Berry, E. (2022, November 19). 101 short exercise quotes to keep you motivated and inspired. Woman's Day. https://www.womansday.com/health-fitness/g2318/healthy-lifestyle-quotes/

Speers, M. (2018, February 16). 12 ways to work out when the only prop you've got is a chair. Weight Watchers. https://www.weightwatchers.com/us/blog/fitness/chair-exercises-for-legs

Stefanacci, R. G. (2022). Changes in the body with aging. MSD Manuals. https://www.msdmanuals.com/home/older-people%E2%80%99s-health-issues/the-aging-body/changes-in-the-body-with-aging

Stein, A. (2020, December 15). Have a seat: Chair yoga provides support and stability. Caregiving. https://chicagocaregiving.com/have-a-seat/

Stump, S. (2016, April 22). World's fittest 96-year-old, Charles Eugster, shares diet and exercise tips. Today. https://www.today.com/health/world-s-fittest-96-year-old-charles-eugster-shares-diet-t87956

Sweat. (2022, December 21). Could SMART fitness goals change the way you train? https://www.sweat.com/blogs/life/goal-setting

10 Benefits of having an active lifestyle for seniors. (n.d.). Northwest Primary Care. https://www.nwpc.com/5-benefits-active-lifestyle-seniors/

The most common causes of limited mobility in seniors. (2022, September 28). Wellness Corner. https://www.hdfcergo.com/health-insurance/wellness-corner/common-causes-for-limited-mobility-in-seniors

30 useful workout log templates (free spreadsheets). (2020, August 18). TemplateArchive.com. https://templatearchive.com/workout-log/

Top 10 benefits seniors experience when exercising. (2022, October 17). Excellence in Fitness. https://www.excellenceinfitness.com/blog/benefits-exercising-seniors

Tricep lifts exercise. (n.d.). More Life Health. https://morelifehealth.com/tricep-lifts

21 chair exercises for seniors: A comprehensive visual guide. (2023, April 13). California Mobility. https://californiamobility.com/21-chair-exercises-for-seniors-visual-guide/#15_heel_slides

Vann, M. R. (2016, August 1). *The 15 most common health concerns for seniors.* Everyday Health. https://www.everydayhealth.com/news/most-common-health-concerns-seniors/

Veras Investments. (2020, November 12). *Seated alternating diagonal reach* [Video]. YouTube. https://www.youtube.com/watch?v=-Qr62kErzWw

Vive Health. (2020, February 2). *Seated jumping jacks chair exercise* [Video]. YouTube. https://www.youtube.com/watch?v=zKZOVD30vKo

Vive Health. (2020, February 5). *Seated tap dance chair exercise* [Video]. YouTube. https://www.youtube.com/watch?v=EinDau-w8AI

Wahome, C. (n.d.). *4 benefits of chair exercises.* WebMD. https://www.webmd.com/fitness-exercise/features/4-benefits-chair-exercises-seniors

Wamsley, L. (2019, April 5). *Such great heights: 84-year-old pole vaulter keeps raising the bar.* NPR. https://www.npr.org/2019/04/05/710417769/such-great-heights-84-year-old-pole-vaulter-keeps-raising-the-bar#:

What are common mobility issues in old age? (n.d.). SonderCare. https://www.sondercare.com/learn/mobility-disability/what-common-mobility-issues-old-age/

Williams, L. (2022, October 21). *11 accessible chair exercises for seniors.* Verywell Fit. https://www.verywellfit.com/chair-exercises-for-seniors-4161267

Made in the USA
Monee, IL
18 November 2024

70477806R00125